Doctors' Decisions and the Cost of Medical Care

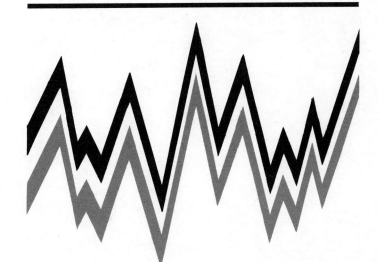

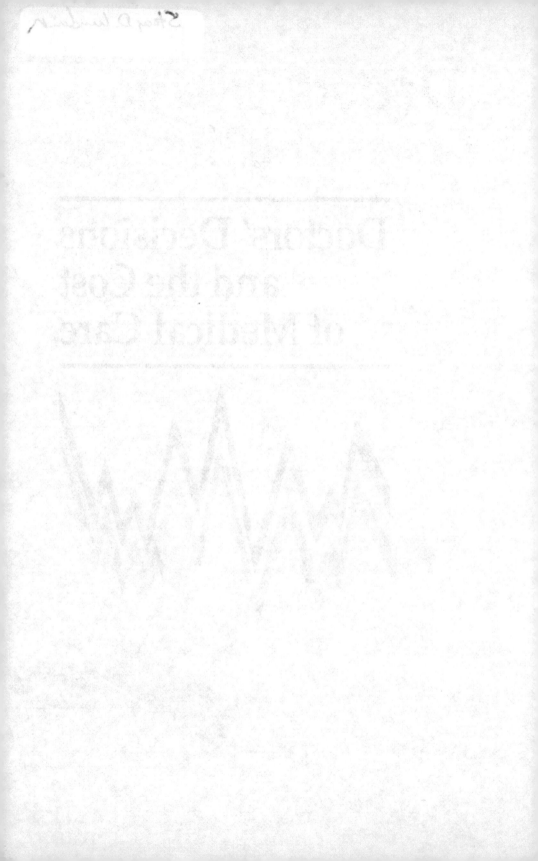

Doctors' Decisions and the Cost of Medical Care

The Reasons for Doctors' Practice Patterns and Ways to Change Them

John M. Eisenberg, M.D.

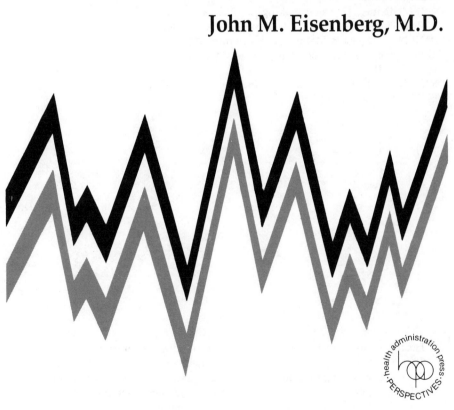

Health Administration Press Perspectives
Ann Arbor, Michigan
1986

Library of Congress Cataloging-in-Publication Data
Eisenberg, John M. (John Mayer), 1946–
   Doctors' decisions and the cost of medical care.

   Bibliography: p.
   Includes index.
   1. Medicine—Decision making. 2. Medical logic.
3. Physicians—Psychology. 4. Medical fees. I. Title.
[DNLM: 1. Decision Making. 2. Economics, Medical.
3. Physicians. 4. Practice Management, Medical.
W 80 E 36d]
R723.5K53 1986   338.4'56161   86–14312
ISBN 0–910701–14–8 (soft)

Health Administration Press
1021 East Huron
Ann Arbor, Michigan 48109
(313) 764-1380

Health Administration Press
Perspectives is an imprint of Health
Administration Press dedicated to
books and other material of timely
and special interest for health
care practitioners.

Contents

List of Figures

Preface

Differences among physicians in their prescription of medical care are reflected in well-documented variations in practice patterns. Many simple single explanations have been put forth to explain these differences, ranging from financial motivation to fear of malpractice and to the uncertainty inherent in medical care. Equally simple proposals to change doctors' practice patterns have been suggested. However, they may be too simple to shed light on why some medical practices need to be changed. Whereas a single intervention such as education or financial penalties may change physicians' practices to some extent, it addresses only one of the motivating forces in doctors' decision making. Unfortunately, most efforts to influence doctors' prescription of services have not been adequately evaluated, so their claims of success can only be accepted as articles of faith.

In truth, a variety of factors influence medical decision making, including physicians' self-interest, their role as patient advocates, and their concern for social good. To alter physicians' practice patterns in an efficient manner, we must understand these influences on decision making and plan interventions to address them.

This book is an introduction to the research that has elucidated the reasons doctors practice the way they do and make the decisions they do. It reviews the complex array of motivations in medical practice and emphasizes that no single simple explanation will suffice. The book also reviews the programs that have been used to change physicians' prescription of medical services, including education, feedback, participation, administrative rules, incentives, and penalties.

Although recent research has elucidated the factors that influence physician utilization of services and has evaluated ways to change that utilization, a number of challenges remain for health services researchers. These include identifying the most efficient ways to improve medical decision making, evaluating sources of data, developing methods to consider the effects of case mix, conducting longitudinal studies, and developing statistical methods to describe utilization patterns.

It is my hope that this book will help both the investigators who carry out this research and those who use their findings. Finally, I hope that the book encourages those who attempt to alter physicians' practices to evaluate whether their interventions work and why.

Acknowledgements

This book is the outgrowth of a paper I was invited to write for a conference sponsored by the National Center for Health Services Research in October 1984: "Planning for the Third Decade of Health Services Research." I am grateful to the Divisions of General Internal Medicine and Health Services Research at Stanford University, where I prepared the paper while on sabbatical. After the conference, the paper was expanded and revised while I was conducting research projects evaluating variations in the use of ancillary services (funded by the Robert Wood Johnson Foundation) and physician decision making (funded by grant HS04953 from the National Center for Health Services Research).

I am especially grateful to two teachers who were most influential in the development of my interest in physicians' practice patterns: Gerald T. Perkoff, M.D., and Samuel P. Martin, M.D. Both men are master clinician-educators and clinician-investigators who turned their attention to health services research in midcareer. They have inspired a generation of physicians to think carefully and critically about the way medical care is provided. Sankey V. Williams, M.D., has been my partner in this work on doctors' practice patterns, and most of the ideas in this book either were shaped by him or were his ideas originally. I am also indebted to the leadership of the Department of Medicine and the School of Medicine at the University of Pennsylvania, who have been supportive of our effort to bridge clinical medicine and health services research. Mr. Sol Katz's generosity has been critical in enabling us to carry out our work.

I also want to thank Nancie Lucera, who has helped to keep this project on track, Michael Bokulich for his editorial advice, and my colleagues who have commented on draft manuscripts. My family—DD, Billy, and Michael—have been wonderfully supportive. Not only have they humored me but they have managed not to trip over any of the piles of papers in the study.

Part I

Understanding Variations in Physicians' Practice Patterns

Physicians serve a dual role in the provision of personal health services. Like the player-manager of an athletic team, the physician is responsible for calling the plays in medical care as well as working with others to carry them out. In the parlance of economics, this dual role means that the physician influences the cost and quality of medical care in two ways: first, by organizing and directing the production process; and second, by providing some of the productive input [1]. Although physicians' fees represent only about 20 percent of health care costs, as much as 80 percent of expenditures for medical care are for services prescribed by physicians [2, 3].

The medical profession may complain that its freedom to prescribe care is being constrained by external forces (such as utilization review, preadmission certification, and second opinion for surgery), but not long ago the inability of many patients to pay for care was even more limiting on medical decision making. The fact that doctors today are being urged to share their decision making with patients and other health professionals bespeaks the central role that the doctor's decision still plays. Even as medical care systems become more complex, with larger group practices, vertically integrated hospital organizations, prepaid plans, and large health care chains, the doctor-patient relationship remains the focus of medical care.

Because of the central economic role of physicians' clinical decisions and their prescriptions for clinical services, it is important to understand the factors that influence medical decision making. Here there is a parallel between research in the biomedical sciences and in health services research. In biomedical research, investigation into the causes of disease and the body's response to drugs provides insights into normal human physiology. In the same way, variation among physicians' practice styles and their responses to efforts to change their behavior can serve as probes to understand why doctors practice the way they do.

Part I of this book reviews the forces that shape the multitude of decisions made in the course of a day's practice, including whether to admit a patient into the hospital, to recommend surgery, to discharge a patient, to order a diagnostic test, or to prescribe a medication.

The emphasis on decision making by physicians is not meant to derogate the importance of patients and their families in determining the course of diagnosis and treatment. Certainly, the patient's values and preferences should be an essential component of decision making in medical care. Nor is the emphasis on doctors' decisions intended to neglect the role of other health professionals in medical decision making. However, because the physician traditionally has been most responsible for decisions about diagnosis and treatment and because most evaluations of medical decision making have studied physicians, it is the decision making of physicians which is emphasized in the following pages.

1

Variation in Medical Decision Making

Doctors do not all practice alike. When one doctor might suggest surgery, another might prefer medical therapy. When one might advise a patient to undergo extensive diagnostic testing, another might suggest observation for a few weeks. That this variation in medical practice exists should surprise no one. Because much of medical knowledge is ambiguous and because few services are absolutely necessary, this variety in clinical practice patterns should be expected.

This variation in medical practice patterns is a demonstration of the fact that the "essentiality argument" of economics is not fulfilled in medical care [4]. Since few medical services are absolutely essential for society's well-being, the use of most of these services is sensitive to changes in the financial resources available to purchase them [5]. In other words, physicians have few iron-clad rules for practicing medicine. The degree to which medical practice varies among physicians has been documented by a number of health services researchers and is quite impressive. This variation is more than a simple statistical artifact; it provides valuable insights into the factors that influence physicians' prescription of services.

Evidence of Variation in Medical Practice

Variation has been observed in all elements of medical practice, including rates of surgery, drug prescription, diagnostic testing, hospitalization, and length of stay. One of the best documented is the regional variation in the proportion of the population who undergo surgery yearly. Studies

of surgical rates in small geographical areas in New England have revealed fourfold differences in hysterectomy rates, sixfold in tonsillectomy
rates, and fourfold in prostatectomy rates [6–9]. Similar variations between small areas have been seen with common surgical procedures in
Wales, Canada, England, and Norway [10–12]. Overall rates of surgery
in the United States exceed those in England [13]. Figure 1.1 is reproduced from the classic study by McPherson and colleagues documenting
international differences in surgery rates. A similar analysis of surgical
rates in small geographic areas has revealed fivefold differences in Manitoba, Canada [14]. Although some differences among regions are inevitable due to differences in the medical care needs of the populations,
such wide variations in surgery rates in Canada cannot be explained by
a "needs model," which relates different rates of surgery to differences in
clinical characteristics of populations [15].

Nonsurgical rates vary even more than surgical rates [16, 17]. For
example, in the state of Washington, studies of hospitalization rates of
children covered by Medicaid showed remarkable variation between different areas [18]. The four diagnostic categories with the highest variability for hospitalization were gastroenteritis (18-fold differences), lower
respiratory tract infections (15-fold differences), upper respiratory tract
infections (8-fold differences), and ear, nose, and throat surgery (6-fold
differences). Similar variation exists among hospitalization rates for diagnosis related groups (DRGs) in 30 hospital market areas in Maine [19].
Whereas hysterectomy rates have been shown to vary 3.5-fold, 80 percent
of DRGs showed even greater variation. Only the rates for three diagnostic
groups (acute myocardial infarction, gastrointestinal hemorrhage, and
cerebrovascular accidents) and six surgical groups were less variable than
rates for hysterectomy.

Although hospitalization and surgical rates are greater in the United
States than in the United Kingdom, the average length of a hospital stay
is shorter in the United States. Abel-Smith has suggested that these differences in length of stay seem to depend on the custom of the treating
doctor and he points out that different countries have different customs
[20]. These differences may result from differences in the organization of
medical care. For example, longer lengths of stay in the United Kingdom,
Sweden, and West Germany than in the United States may result from
the greater ability of the American primary care physician to admit patients to the hospital. Early discharge policies depend on the confidence
of the doctor responsible for hospital care that the patient will receive
proper treatment after discharge. This confidence, in turn, depends on
whether the same doctor is responsible for both hospital and primary

Figure 1.1   International differences in surgical rates. Mean and range
of age- and sex-standardized rates for common surgical
procedures in New England, Norway, and the West
Midlands.

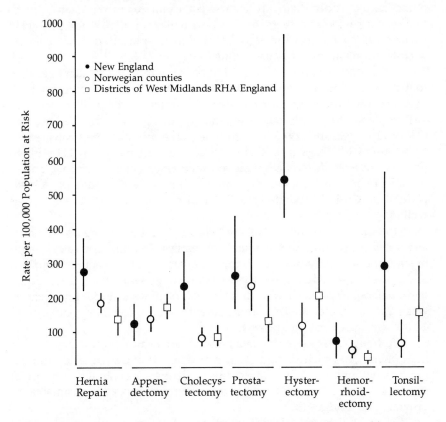

Source: McPherson, K., J.E. Wennberg, O.B. Hovind, et al. [10]. Reprinted by permission of *The New England Journal of Medicine*, 1982; 307:1312.

care (as often is the case in the United States) or whether there is good
communication between the hospital and the primary care system.

In addition to these substantial international and interregional differences in surgical and hospitalization rates and lengths of stay [21],
intraregional variations among hospitals have also been well documented. For example, sizeable variations exist in cesarian section rates
among hospitals in California [22]. In addition, different hospitals provide substantially different services to surgical patients [23]. A recent
study by the Office of Technology Assessment has reviewed the wide

variations in length of stay among hospitals and has shown that the differences could not be explained by clinical information [24].

Studies of variation in medical care have revealed that not only are differences found among regions and hospitals, but they can also be found among individual physicians. For example, in one state, practitioners vary widely in their rates of hospitalization [25]. Wide physician variation is also seen in rates of admission to special hospital services, such as neonatal intensive care units [26].

Once patients are hospitalized or have surgery, the ancillary services that their doctors prescribe will also vary. This can be shown for both inpatient and outpatient practice. Variation in the use of ancillary services such as laboratory tests has been shown among regions [27], hospitals [28], and physicians [29–33], even when case mix has been considered. Prescription of drugs also varies by region and physician [34–40]. In England, fivefold differences were recorded among eight hospitals in their use of preoperative chest radiography. This variation could not be explained on clinical grounds [41]. Rates of referral to consultants vary as well [42].

International comparisons are helpful in analyzing the use of ancillary services and suggest remarkable differences in utilization rates, length of stay, and surgical rates. For example, Epstein and colleagues compared ambulatory test ordering for hypertensive patients in the United States and England [43]. They found that for each of 13 tests studied, utilization was equal or higher for American patients, with differences being up to 41-fold (for electrocardiography).

Although less data are available about health professionals other than physicians, such as dentists or nurse practitioners, variation in their practice patterns is likely. One study of dentists has shown substantial variation in rates of performing three restorative procedures: amalgams, crowns, and bridges [44].

Most of these studies have attempted to control for the fact that different doctors and different hospitals care for different types of patients. In some studies, apparent differences in utilization disappear when the types of patients being cared for are held constant [45–47]. Becker and Sloan have demonstrated that differences in case mix are important in explaining variations among hospitals in length of stay, diagnostic tests, and consultations [48]. Unfortunately, the ability of researchers to determine confounding variables, such as the severity of disease, the types and severity of coexisting illnesses, and the degree of disability caused by an illness, is limited in almost all these studies of variation. When claims forms are used to characterize physicians' practice patterns, the advantage of studying large numbers of clinical encounters is offset by limited information for each encounter. Chart reviews would provide more information, but at substantially greater cost to the researcher.

Recent reviews have summarized this convincing evidence of substantial variation among regions, small areas, hospitals, and practitioners for the entire array of medical care services [49–53]. A special issue of the journal *Health Affairs* (Summer 1984) emphasized the importance of these variations in the utilization of medical services, and one article suggested the potential of this information for changing utilization rates [54].

The implications of variation in medical care have been further publicized by testimony before Congressional committees [55] and by articles in the lay press. For example, Bunker's review in the April 25, 1985 issue of *The New York Review of Books*, entitled "When Doctors Disagree," suggests that variation in physicians' practice styles is one cause of inefficiency in medical care [56]. He proposes that if a national program to assess medical technology were established and if doctors were taught to base their decisions on reliable evidence, the need to ration medical care could be avoided. For a different audience, the business community, Caper and Zubkoff have argued that analysis of the rates and patterns of medical care within small areas can be a powerful technique for identifying discretionary services [57]. By this technique, opportunities for savings in employers' health insurance budgets may be found. Caper and Zubkoff suggest that when utilization rates are high, the number of marginally indicated services will be greater.

Variation, Quality, and the Necessity of Medical Care

Although revelation of these differences among physicians, hospitals, and areas in the utilization of medical care has made the headlines, variations in the consumption of most other economic goods and services would probably attract little attention. Would anyone be surprised by wide differences among regions in the amount spent on meals in restaurants or on automobiles? Why then has so much concern been focused on variation in medical care utilization? One reason is that most medical care bills are paid by third-party payers, so unusually high expenses by one person are paid by all those who share in the pooled costs incurred by the payer. Second, medical care is generally considered to be a need, not a luxury such as a restaurant meal or a fancy car. Variation should be caused, the argument goes, by unavoidable illness rather than by doctors' habits or consumers' preferences. Given the pooled responsibility for paying for medical care, cost should be balanced by benefits in improved health. In addition to this cost-benefit tradeoff, the risk-benefit tradeoff must be considered. Variation in medical care utilization suggests that some patients are receiving medical care when the benefits of care may be less than the risk of adverse side effects from treatment.

However, the fact that variation exists does not necessarily mean that unnecessary services are being provided. Few studies support the usual assumption that lower levels of utilization represent a more desirable level of care. In fact, one study found no relationship between high utilization rates and overtreatment in a focused review of dental utilization [58].

Despite the lack of support for a close relationship between high utilization and unnecessary utilization, substantial evidence shows that overuse does occur in most areas of medical practice [59–62]. One area of practice in which unnecessary use has been documented is the ordering of diagnostic tests [63–68]. For example, at one teaching hospital up to 65 percent of the orders for selected laboratory tests, 30 percent of stat orders, 11 percent of chest radiographic examinations, and 26 percent of nursing services were judged to be clinically unnecessary [69]. At another teaching hospital, between 26 and 43 percent of laboratory tests were considered unnecessary when medical records were audited. At still another, about half of patients who had repeated determinations with the same test were judged to have undergone unnecessary testing [70].

Unfortunately, few studies are available on the appropriateness of diagnostic testing at nonteaching hospitals. In one health maintenance organization, careful review of the indications for diagnostic radiography revealed that unnecessary services were being provided. The utilization of diagnostic radiographic examinations of the skull, chest, and upper gastrointestinal tract could have been reduced substantially without significantly altering the diagnosis, treatment, or outcome for most patients, with a resultant decrease in radiation exposure to patients and in costs for diagnostic medical care [71].

Similar evidence shows unnecessary care in other areas. Unnecessary prescriptions have been well documented, including excessive doses, inappropriate drugs, excessive injections, and the use of more expensive brands [72–75]. These unnecessary prescriptions are not only costly but potentially harmful to the patient [76, 77]. As much as 25 percent of days of hospital care and about 20 percent of surgical procedures have been considered inappropriate [78, 79]. About 30 percent of restorative dentistry has been judged to be unnecessary by a panel of consultants [80]. In addition to the use and choice of procedures and days of hospitalization, physicians can influence the intensity of nursing care provided to inpatients. One study found that physicians at a major teaching hospital gave excessive orders for nursing care (such as checking vital signs and fluid balance) [81].

In the Office of Technology Assessment review of variations in length of stay for patients with selected diagnoses, Chassin reported that shorter hospital stays were not found to be harmful [82]. In fact, all of the studies he reviewed concluded that short lengths of stay could be employed on an experimental basis with safety. However, Chassin cautions against uncritical adoption of these conclusions, largely because of the lack of statistical power in research studies to detect clinically significant increases in morbidity or mortality. The literature reviewed also failed to shed additional light on the meaning of regional variations in length of stay.

Therefore, the challenge in understanding the practice patterns of physicians is not only to document that variation exists. To consider only the extent of variation assumes that attention need only be focused on those physicians whose practice profiles are exceptionally high or low— the doctors whose practices are statistical outliers. The documentation of substantial unnecessary prescription of medical care does not per se suggest this. Reducing variation in medical practice is not necessarily an appropriate goal. Such a policy may only cause physicians to provide similar amounts of unnecessary services or to deny similar amounts of necessary care. In our attention to the possible overuse of medical care by physicians and hospitals or in areas that have high rates of use, we must remember the converse—that low rates may suggest underuse. Just as important as the variability in rates of use that characterize outliers is the possibility that the standard of care from which the outliers deviate may be inappropriate. Often the problem may not be a few providers who are practicing in an unusual manner; the problem may be that the mode of practice needs to be altered.

However, if the variation in utilization of services does reflect the prescription of unnecessary care, then reducing variation will serve an end more fruitful than simply searching for homogeneity. It will enable the medical profession to identify and eliminate unnecessary care that is costly and potentially harmful.

Because unnecessary medical care may be harmful as well as wasteful, several investigators have evaluated the relationship between variation and the outcomes of medical care. For example, studies of surgical outcome have consistently shown an inverse relationship between the volume of surgery and mortality rates as well as other outcomes, such as infection. These data suggest an association between high rates of utilization and better surgical outcomes. Whereas higher utilization could produce practitioners with more experience and therefore better outcomes, it is also possible that better outcomes attract more patients or that higher rates of utilization reflect a lower threshold for treatment, thus including lower-risk patients [83].

Reasons for Variation

In addition to simply documenting the variation in rates of surgery, hospitalization, and diagnostic testing and their relation to variation in outcomes, we must understand the underlying factors that influence medical practice. For example, regions with high per-capita admission rates for diabetes mellitus are those in which physicians' criteria for admission are less stringent [84]. Why are their criteria for hospitalizing diabetic patients different from those of other doctors? Since physicians are responsible for the decisions to admit, test, and treat that generate these differences in utilization, it follows that the solution of this mystery will require that the factors influencing medical decision making be understood.

Data about variations in medical practice can be used not only to monitor variation in utilization and outcomes but also to identify areas in which the education of physicians might decrease variation. The data on differences among physicians' practice patterns offer clues about the process of medical decision making and the factors influencing this process. Medical decision making is admittedly complex and efforts to open the "black box" of medical judgement must involve a variety of perspectives, including clinical, economic, psychological, and sociological. Without understanding why medical practice has such wide variation, it will be difficult—and perhaps impossible—to alter this practice effectively.

The reasons for unnecessary services are many, as casual conversation with any practicing physician will reveal [85, 86]. A model of physician behavior that does not consider the complex interaction of influences—the supply of hospitals and of physicians, economic inducement, style of practice, physician characteristics, character of the practice setting, influence of clinical leaders, concern for the patient's well-being, patient demand and other patient characteristics, and the perceived good of society—oversimplifies the challenge of understanding and changing practice patterns of physicians.

An Early Hypothesis: Supply Breeds Demand

Among the factors that influence physician practice patterns, one of the first to be recognized was the supply of hospital beds. Popularized as "Roemer's law," the usual explanation for the frequently observed correlation between hospitalization rates and the number of hospital beds in a community is that the need for services expands to fill the available supply [87, 88].

Recent evidence for the effect of empty hospital beds on admission rates has been provided by an analysis showing the association of low hospital occupancy rates with higher rates of hospitalization when other factors were controlled [89]. Conversely, utilization may decrease when beds are full. For example, a study of urban hospitals in Manitoba, Canada, found that inpatient surgical procedures and admissions decreased while overall occupancy rates increased from 80 percent to 85 percent [90]. The increase in occupancy rates was also coincident with the opening of a special outpatient surgery unit in one of Winnipeg's teaching hospitals. Outpatient surgery increased but average surgical workloads showed little change.

Another change that occurred in Manitoba at this time weakens the argument that inpatient surgery decreased in response to a tighter bed supply and the availability of an outpatient surgical unit. This change was that general practitioners recently entering urban practice had increasing difficulties in obtaining admitting privileges. These practitioners were likely to begin by working in emergency rooms and doing outpatient surgery. However, even where this change was seen, an overall increase in outpatient surgery occurred, suggesting increased activity among surgically active physicians who were already established [91].

In another study, when the availability of intensive care beds became limited, fewer patients were admitted with chest pain and a higher percentage of admitted patients actually had suffered an acute myocardial infarction [92]. This percentage increased linearly with the restriction in bed capacity. These three studies suggest that physicians systematically raise their threshold for admitting patients when beds are less available. Therefore, the availability of beds does seem to influence their clinical decision making.

Despite this evidence confirming the "availability effect" of hospital beds on admission rates, Pauly found that the supply of beds was only weakly related to hospitalization rates [93]. Similarly, in one study, admission rates for children covered by Medicaid were not related to hospital bed supply or occupancy [94]. In addition, no relationship was seen between the availability of hospital beds and hysterectomy rates in Manitoba [95].

Because the studies that did show an effect of bed supply on hospitalization rates often involved situations in which beds were actually in short supply, the conflicting findings may be because the relationship between bed supply and hospitalization rates holds more strongly in a narrow range of occupancy. For example, occupancy rates of 60 percent versus 70 percent may show little difference in their effect on doctors' decisions, but an occupancy of 85 or 90 percent may affect them differently. This may be because a high occupancy rate makes it difficult to find a bed on an appropriate service on a specific day or because physicians may be induced to be more hesitant to admit patients, perhaps due to a group ethos about leaving some beds available for emergencies and severely ill patients. Alternatively, hospital administrators and medical staff leaders might encourage doctors to admit patients more readily when the hospital's occupancy is down, whether it be 60 or 70 percent occupancy.

The argument that the need for hospitalization expands to fill the supply of hospital beds is parallel to the argument of the "technological imperative," according to which the mere availability of biomedical technology induces its use [96]. This principle has been invoked to explain why physicians might order a new diagnostic test even if its potential contribution to clinical care is small.

Although the technological imperative may exist and the availability effect of hospital beds may exist, neither fully explains physician behavior. Neither is an effective model for understanding why doctors would fill empty beds or prescribe new diagnostic tests unless doing so has some potential value to the patient, physician, or society at large. Although the possibility of an availability effect or technological imperative may scratch the surface of the black box of physician behavior, they do little to offer a satisfactory explanation for variation or overuse of medical services.

Another proposed explanation for variation in the rates of medical services is the number of physicians. Most studies focus on the link between surgical rates and the supply of surgeons. In 1970, Bunker demonstrated the relationship between the rate of surgery and the number of surgeons per capita [97]. Other studies have reached similar conclusions—that the availability of surgeons creates the demand for more surgery [98–102]. However, as is the case with the argument for the availability effect of hospital beds, evidence about the effect of physician supply on utilization is conflicting [103]. For 1968, 1969, and 1971, an association was seen between the number of surgeons in the Canadian provinces and their surgical rates, but in a 10-year analysis for 1968 to 1977, no statistical associations were found [104]. In another study, no relationship was seen in Manitoba between hysterectomy rates and physician supply [105]. Similarly, in the United States, there was little consistent or significant effect of the supply of surgeons on rates of inpatient surgery [106].

Studies investigating the effect of the supply of physicians on the volume of services other than surgery have also reached conflicting conclusions. Although some evidence indicates that the supply of nonsurgical physicians influences the use of diagnostic tests [107, 108], another study has found no effect of the physician-to-population ratio on test use [109]. The same study that found a correlation between the supply of surgeons and the frequency of surgery for children covered by Medicaid did not find a similar relationship between the supply of physicians and admission rates [110]. On the other hand, Rossiter and Wilensky did find that the number of physician visits increases with an increase in the physician-to-population ratio [111].

Although proof of an availability effect of physician supply on resource use in medical care remains indefinite, it is interesting in retrospect that Fuchs and Kramer warned, in 1972 when the nation was priming the pump of medical education to produce more physicians, that "we should be wary of plans which assume that the cost of medical care would be reduced by increasing the supply of physicians" [112]. Even now that the pump has been primed so much that the supply is overflowing, the effect that a surplus of physicians has on the volume of services is not yet clear, although most investigators suggest that utilization will increase.

Can Physicians Induce Demand?

In addition to studying the statistical relationships between the availability of hospital beds or physician supply and medical care utilization, health care researchers have sought other evidence that physicians induce demand for their services. Like the literature on physician and hospital supply, most of this literature has been based on aggregate data and has drawn conclusions from correlations in cross-sectional data. Little longitudinal research has been done. Wilensky and Rossiter have summarized the methodological problems with the use of cross-sectional data to determine the relative importance of physician-induced demand: 1) these data ignore characteristics of the area, such as tastes, income, incidence of illness, and insurance coverage; 2) the data ignore the potential problem of border-crossing patients (those living in one area who seek care from providers in another area) which produces bias in the operational physician-to-population ratio in the service area; 3) equal weight is attached to each observation regardless of the size of the market that the observations reflect; and 4) the data assume that the areas being studied are representative of medical practice in general [113].

Although the idea of physician-induced demand is certainly not new to health economics [114–117], four studies published in 1983 offer valuable insights into its importance and the way it operates. Rossiter and Wilensky used data from the National Medical Care Expenditure Survey in two reports to assess the role of physician-initiated demand [118, 119]. Information was collected in the Survey for 1977 from a sample of 40,000 individuals representative of the U.S. population. Because the data could be disaggregated, the authors were able to be more specific in the questions they investigated than had been possible previously with aggregate data. In addition, the Survey had asked patients whether a visit had been made by appointment and, if so, whether the physician had suggested the visit. Rossiter and Wilensky found that 39 percent of ambulatory visits to physicians and 43 percent of all visits (inpatient and outpatient) in 1977 were initiated by the physician (1.5 visits per person per year). The remainder were initiated by patients. They also showed that a higher physician-to-population ratio was, in fact, associated with more visits and that these visits were physician initiated. However, the magnitude of this increase in visits that was related to the supply of physicians was small, with the elasticity being about 6 percent. The role of the physician in inducing demand for medical care due to an increased physician supply was substantially less than the role played by the patient's health. These findings are consistent with the notion that some physician inducement does occur, particularly in cases where physician discretion is greater (that is, ambulatory care and ancillary services including radiographs and laboratory tests).

A third study published in 1983 also found evidence for physician inducement [120]. Between 1976 and 1977, Colorado's Medicare reimbursement system changed, resulting in a large increase in some physicians' reimbursement rates and a relative decrease in others. Rice found that declining reimbursement rates resulted in the provision of more intensive services (both in terms of the quantity of services and their level of complexity) and that increasing reimbursement rates resulted in less intensive services. This relationship was true of surgical services but not of medical follow-up visits. It was also true of laboratory tests but not radiology services. These results suggest that physicians provide different intensities of care depending on the need to recoup lost income when their reimbursement changes.

Finally, Roos found that when new general practitioners (some of whom did surgery) moved into rural areas in Canada, surgical utilization increased by 17 percent [121]. When a surgically active physician left an area, however, two important trends resulted. Overall surgical utilization for the population remained the same, but the surgical workloads of the remaining physicians increased by 18.7 percent. Therefore, although Rice suggests that physicians' prescription of medical services is responsive in both directions [122], Roos suggests that physicians are more likely to increase rather than decrease the volume of services they prescribe in response to changes in supply or other economic factors [123].

Because of the limitations of the cross-sectional aggregate data used in these studies, especially in discerning the motivation for medical decisions, Hemenway and Fallon used hypothetical cases to determine whether physicians practice differently in areas with different physician-to-population ratios [124]. Their results are consistent with the theory of induced demand. Physician density was positively and significantly correlated with aggressiveness of treatment. Their regression equations suggest that a physician from an area with a low density of physicians such as Portland, Maine, has a 23 percent likelihood of recommending aggressive treatment, whereas an otherwise identical doctor practicing in the very-high-density Boston area has a 45 percent chance of advocating aggressive treatment. In addition, doctors with high incomes tend to be more aggressive. Hemenway and Fallon suggest that this demand inducement could be related both to doctors having more time to do what they believe useful and to financial considerations that increase the ease with which they can rationalize to themselves the need for more intensive treatment. Although other factors such as the role of teaching hospitals, group practice, and patient preferences were not evaluated in this study of simulated cases, the results do suggest that some differences in medical decision making may be due to demographic factors such as physician density.

Not all services that are initiated by a physician are necessarily induced by the physician. Wilensky and Rossiter have attempted to clarify this distinction by defining physician-induced demand as that which occurs when services are recommended above and beyond what a patient would be willing to purchase if the patient knew as much as the physician [125, 126]. Of course, the services that patients would be willing to purchase are not necessarily those that are medically appropriate or those that would have a favorable effect on their health. Nonetheless, this definition of physician-induced demand does suggest that part of doctors' decision making reflects their acting on behalf of their patients and carrying out their patients' wishes (at least the doctor's perception of the patient's wishes). Beyond this, physicians may prescribe some services that a well-informed patient would not want. These are the services that are induced by the physician. The model that Wilensky and Rossiter present suggests that physicians initiate most medical care and that this physician-initiated care is the sum of care that patients would choose and would not choose (the latter being physician induced).

Therefore, only part of physician-initiated demand is actually physician induced. The rest may be suggested by the physician but would have been chosen by the patient as well. Wilensky and Rossiter recognize that physician-initiated demand is more easily measured than physician-induced demand, because consumer preferences are difficult to measure. Nonetheless, from the perspective of understanding physician decision making, it is helpful to understand that a large part of medical care is initiated by physicians and that some of that care is physician induced. Although Wilensky and Rossiter argue that the amount of physician-induced demand is small, they estimate that 90 percent of health care costs are physician initiated.

What Motivates Medical Demand?

The demonstration of variation in practice patterns, the evidence of over-utilization, and the suggestion of a relationship (albeit inconsistent) between hospital and physician supply and utilization all imply that the medical care system may generate activity for itself. While this may be the case, it leaves open the question why. The implications for public policy would be quite different if this increased activity were a response to an unmet public desire for more medical care than if it were the result of a desire by providers to increase their practice volume for economic or other self-motivated reasons.

To understand physicians' practice behavior better, we must investigate factors that influence clinical decision making by physicians. Why do physicians decide to prescribe medical services, whether hospitalization, surgery, diagnostic tests, or drugs? A number of forces on medical decision making have been described. These forces demonstrate the complexity of the influences on physicians' utilization of services. Some relate to the physicians' economic self-interest, personal style, and practice environment. These factors can be described as those related to the self-fulfilling physician. Other influences relate to the physician's role as the patient's agent, as a patient advocate whose decisions are driven by a well-meaning desire to act on behalf of the patient's physical or economic health and the patient's preferences. Still other influences suggest that the physician's decision making is guided by a desire to provide the most good to the most people, a principle of maximizing the social benefit of medical care.

Thresholds in Decision Making

Whether the physician is considering his or her own well-being, that of the patient, or that of society as a whole, medical decision making can be characterized by the use of thresholds for prescribing medical services [127, 128]. The threshold is the level above which the probability of disease causes a physician to take a certain action, such as ordering a test, prescribing a medication, or recommending surgery. Below that probability, the physician may take other actions, each of which has its own threshold. Understanding physicians' thresholds may help to explain the variation in their prescription of medical services.

Figure 1.2 illustrates the threshold concept by showing a bar that represents the range of probabilities that a patient has a disease, ranging from 0 percent to 100 percent. At some low probability of disease, the physician will take no action but may, for example, reassure the patient. The threshold for testing (that is, the probability above which testing would be ordered) usually lies below the threshold for treatment. The latter is called the test-treatment threshold, because it is the probability above which the doctor will change his decision from testing to treating. Therefore, the physician may choose to test a patient for whom a disease is suspected if the perceived probability is both too high to do nothing and too low to initiate treatment without more information. If the test results cause the physician to revise the probability upward and if the revised probability exceeds the threshold for a particular treatment, the physician will prescribe the treatment.

The thresholds that the physician chooses for testing and treatment are based on the perception of the benefits and costs involved. In the medical sense, the benefits include the potential reduction in morbidity

Figure 1.2 Thresholds for testing and treatment.

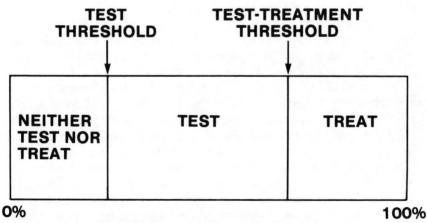

or mortality from testing and treatment. The costs include the risk and economic cost of the medical service, including potential side effects. The relationship between the threshold (T) and the benefits (B) and costs (C) of the contemplated action can be described as follows:

$T = 1 / (1 + B / C)$.

It follows from this relationship that the threshold for testing or treatment will be very low if the benefits are substantially larger than the costs. This situation would result in the benefit-to-cost ratio being large and the denominator of the threshold equation being large, thereby resulting in a small fraction. Hence, the threshold will be low. Conversely, the threshold will be very high if the costs are substantially larger than the benefits. In this situation, the benefit-to-cost ratio would be small and the denominator of the threshold equation would be close to the value of one. As a result, the threshold would be close to one as well, representing a threshold probability that approaches 100 percent. In other words, the doctor would not take the action (be it testing or treatment) unless the probability of the patient having the disease in question was quite high.

Therefore, the threshold model of medical decision making explains how clinical characteristics of the situation (for example, probability, clinical risks, and benefits) and the economic cost of the action should influence the probability at which a doctor prescribes a test or treatment. The threshold for action will range between zero and one (or 0 percent and 100 percent) depending on the relationship between the benefits and costs (including risks) of the contemplated medical action. Used in this way, the threshold is a normative concept. However, it can be expanded to describe medical decision making as well [129].

As the literature on physician variation and physician-induced demand implies, medical decision making is a function of more influences than simply clinical data. The benefits and costs that a physician considers will certainly include the possible clinical benefits for the patient, but they will probably also include the benefits and costs of the action to the physician and to society as a whole. Therefore, the physician's threshold for action will be based on a complex combination of the perceived probability of disease; the potential clinical benefit to the patient; the potential clinical risks to the patient; the cost to the patient; the economic benefit to the physician and his practice organization; the potential benefit or cost to the physician in his satisfaction with his practice; the potential impact on the physician's self-image or status in the community; and the potential benefits, risks, and economic costs to society. The physician will seek to maximize the combined value of these factors. In the language of the decision sciences, the task is a multiattribute utility problem. Not only do physicians need to estimate the value of each variable, but they must weigh the relative importance of each. Doctors will need to make tradeoffs between their own income, the cost to the patient, the pleasure they take in their work, their leisure time, society's limited resources, and the potential benefit of their action for the patient's health.

According to this model of medical decision making, the physician will weigh this panoply of considerations, decide on what the threshold for action should be, compare it with the estimate of the probability of disease for the individual patient, and make a decision. The challenge to the researcher and policy maker alike is to observe this complex decision-making process and to derive from it the influence of these various factors. By observing how doctors make their decisions, we may be able to discern the reasons for the way they practice, whether it be the influence of personal income, the ability to estimate the likelihood of disease, or the willingness to consider the patients' own values.

In the following pages, I review the evidence that these factors influence the decisions made by practicing physicians. The factors can be described in three sets: the physician's own interests and desires, the patient's benefit, and the benefit to society at large.

References

1. Pauly, M.V. *Doctors and Their Workshops.* Chicago: National Bureau of Economic Research, The University of Chicago Press, 1980.

2. Gibson, R.M., D.R. Waldo, and K.R. Levit. National health expenditures, 1982. *Health Care Financing Rev.* 1983; 5:1–30.

3. Wilensky, G.R., and L.F. Rossiter. The relative importance of physician-induced demand for medical care. *Milbank Mem. Fund Q.* 1983; 61:252–77.

4. Fuchs, V.R., and M.J. Kramer. *Determinants of Expenditures for Physicians' Services in the United States 1948–68.* Washington, D.C.: National Center for Health Services Research and Development, Department of Health Education and Welfare, December 1972; 1–63. DHEW publication no. (HSM) 73–3013.

5. Roos, L.L., Jr., N.P. Roos, S.M. Cageorge, and J.P. Nicol. How good are the data: Reliability of one health care data bank. *Med. Care.* 1982; 20:266–76.

6. Wennberg, J.E., and A. Gittelsohn. Small area variations in health care delivery. *Science.* 1973; 182:1102–8.

7. Wennberg, J.E., and A. Gittelsohn. Health care delivery in Maine: I. Patterns of use of common surgical procedures. *J. Maine Med. Assoc.* 1975; 66:123–30, 149.

8. Wennberg, J.E., B.A. Barnes, and M. Zubkoff. Professional uncertainty and the problem of supplier-induced demand. *Soc. Sci. Med.* 1982; 16:811–24.

9. Wennberg, J.E., and A. Gittelsohn. Variations in medical care among small areas. *Sci. Am.* 1982; 246(4):120–34.

10. McPherson, K., J.E. Wennberg, O.B. Hovind, and P. Clifford. Small-area variations in the use of common surgical procedures: An international comparison of New England, England, and Norway. *N. Engl. J. Med.* 1982; 307:1310–14.

11. McPherson, K., P.M. Strong, A. Epstein, and L. Jones. Regional variations in the use of common surgical procedures; within and between England and Wales, Canada and the United States of America. *Soc. Sci. Med.* 1981; 15A:273–88.

12. Vayda, E. A comparison of surgical rates in Canada and in England and Wales. *N. Engl. J. Med.* 1973; 289:1224–29.

13. Bunker, J.P. Surgical manpower: A comparison of operations and surgeons in the United States and in England and Wales. *N. Engl. J. Med.* 1970; 282:135–44.

14. Roos, N.P. Hysterectomy: Variation in rates across small areas and across physicians' practices. *Am. J. Public Health.* 1984; 74:327–35.

15. Roos, N.P., and L.L. Roos, Jr. Surgical rate variations: Do they reflect the health or socioeconomic characteristics of the populations? *Med. Care.* 1982; 20:945–58.

16. Blumberg, M.S. Regional differences in hospital use standardized by reported morbidity. *Med. Care.* 1982; 20:931–44.

17. Gornick, M. Medicare patients: Geographic differences in hospital discharge rates and multiple stays. *Soc. Secur. Bull.* 1977; (June):1–20.

18. Connell, F.A., R.W. Day, and J.P. LoGerfo. Hospitalization of Medicaid children: Analysis of small area variations in admission rates. *Am. J. Public Health.* 1981; 71:606–13.

19. Wennberg, J.E., K. McPherson, and P. Caper. Will payment based on diagnosis-related groups control hospital costs? *N. Engl. J. Med.* 1984; 311:295–300.

20. Abel-Smith, B. *Cost Containment in Health Care: A Study of 12 European Countries, 1977–1983.* London: Bedford Square Press of the National Council for Voluntary Organizations, 1984. Occasional Papers on Social Administration, No. 73.

21. Rothberg, D.L. Regional variations in hospital use: Introduction and overview. In Rothberg, D.L., ed. *Regional Variations in Hospital Use.* Lexington, Mass.: Lexington Books, 1982; 1–20.

22. Williams, R.L., and P.M. Chen. Controlling the rise in cesarean section rates by the dissemination of information from vital records. *Am. J. Public Health.* 1983; 73:863–67.

23. Eastaugh, S.R. Cost of elective surgery and utilization of ancillary services in teaching hospitals. *Health Serv. Res.* 1979; 14:290–308.

24. Chassin, M.R. *Variations in Hospital Length of Stay: Their Relationship to Health Outcomes.* Washington, D.C.: Office of Technology Assessment, Congress of the United States; August 1983.

25. Rosenblatt, R.A., and I.S. Moscovice. The physician as gatekeeper: Determinants of physicians' hospitalization rates. *Med. Care.* 1984; 22:150–59.

26. Campbell, D.M. Why do physicians in neonatal care units differ in their admission thresholds? *Soc. Sci. Med.* 1984; 18:365–74.

27. Roos, L.L. Issues in studying ancillary services. *Soc. Sci. Med.* 1982; 16:1583–90.

28. DesHarnais, S., N.M. Kibe, and S. Barbus. Blue Cross and Blue Shield of Michigan Hospital Laboratory On-Site Review Project. *Inquiry.* 1983; 20:328–33.

29. Daniels, M., and S.A. Schroeder. Variation among physicians in use of laboratory tests: II. Relation to clinical productivity and outcomes of care. *Med. Care.* 1977; 15:482–87.

30. Schroeder, S.A., A. Schliftman, and T.E. Piemme. Variation among physicians in use of laboratory tests: Relation to quality of care. *Med. Care.* 1974; 12:709–13.

31. Eisenberg, J.M., and D. Nicklin. Use of diagnostic services by physicians in community practice. *Med. Care.* 1981; 19:297–309.

32. Read, J.L., R.S. Stern, L.A. Thibodeau, D.E. Geer, Jr., and H. Klapholz. Variation in antenatal testing over time and between clinic settings. *J.A.M.A.* 1983; 249:1605–9.

33. Greenwald, H.P., M.L. Peterson, L.P. Garrison, et al. Interspecialty variation in office-based care. *Med. Care.* 1984; 22:14–29.

34. Hartzema, A.G., and D.B. Christensen. Nonmedical factors associated with the prescribing volume among family practitioners in an HMO. *Med. Care.* 1983; 21:990–1000.

35. Dunlop, D.M., R.S. Inch, and J. Paul. A survey of prescribing in Scotland in 1951. *Br. Med. J.* 1953; 1:694–97.

36. Wilson, C.W., J.A. Banks, R.E. Mapes, and S.M. Korte. Pattern of prescribing in general practice. *Br. Med. J.* 1963; 2:604–7.

37. Lee, J.A. Prescribing and other aspects of general practice in three towns. *Proc. R. Soc. Med.* 1964; 57:1041–43.

38. Lee, J.A., P.A. Draper, and M. Weatherall. Prescribing in three English towns. *Milbank Mem. Fund Q.* 1965; 43:285–90.

39. Stolley, P.D., M.H. Becker, L. Lasagna, J.D. McEvilla, and L.M. Sloane. The relationship between physician characteristics and prescribing appropriateness. *Med. Care.* 1972; 10:17–28.

40. Schroeder, S.A., K. Kenders, J.K. Cooper, and T.E. Piemme. Use of laboratory tests and pharmaceuticals: Variation among physicians and effect of cost audit on subsequent use. *J.A.M.A.* 1973; 225:969–73.

41. Royal College of Radiologists. Preoperative chest radiography. *Lancet.* 1979; 2:83–86.

42. Rothert, M.L., D.R. Rovner, A.S. Elstein, G.B. Holzman, M.M. Holmes, and M.M. Ravitch. Differences in medical referral decisions for obesity among family practitioners, general internists, and gynecologists. *Med. Care.* 1984; 22:42–55.

43. Epstein, A.M., R.M. Hartley, J.R. Charlton, et al. A comparison of ambulatory test ordering for hypertensive patients in the United States and England. *J.A.M.A.* 1984; 252:1723–26.

44. Bailit, H.L., J.A. Balzer, and J. Clive. Evaluation of focused dental utilization review system. *Med. Care.* 1983; 21:473–85.

45. See reference 31 above.

46. Lion, J. Case-mix differences among ambulatory patients seen by internists in various settings. *Health Serv. Res.* 1981; 16:407–13.

47. Gold, M. Effects of hospital-based primary care setting on internists' treatment of primary care episodes. *Health Serv. Res.* 1981; 16:383–405.

48. Becker, E.R., and F.A. Sloan. Utilization of hospital services: The roles of teaching, case-mix, and reimbursement. *Inquiry.* 1983; 20:248–57.

49. See reference 15 above.

50. Vayda, E., and W.R. Mindell. Variations in operative rates: What do they mean? *Surg. Clin. North Am.* 1982; 62:627–39.

51. Fineberg, H.V., A.R. Funkhouser, and H. Marks. Variation in medical practice: A review of the literature. Presented at the Conference on Cost-Effective Medical Care: Implications of Variation in Medical Practice, Institute of Medicine, National Academy of Sciences, Washington, D.C., February 1983.

52. Luft, H.S. Variations in clinical practice patterns. *Arch. Intern. Med.* 1983; 143:1861–62.

53. Estes, E.H., Jr. The behavior of health professionals: Impact on cost and quality of care. *Duke Univ. Med. Cent. Perspect.* 1983; 3:7–13.

54. Wennberg, J.E. Dealing with medical practice variations: A proposal for action. *Health Aff.* 1984; 3:6–32.

55. Wennberg, J.E. Testimony before Senate Committee on Appropriations, Subcommittee on Labor, Health and Human Services, and Education; 19 November 1984.

56. Bunker, J.P. When doctors disagree. *N.Y. Rev. Books.* 1985; 32(7):8–12.

57. Caper, P., and M. Zubkoff. Managing medical costs through small area analysis. *Bus. Health.* 1984 September 20; 20–25.

58. See reference 44 above.

59. Griner, P.F., and R.J. Glaser. Misuse of laboratory tests and diagnostic procedures. *N. Engl. J. Med.* 1982; 307:1336–39.

60. Wyszewianski, L., J.R.C. Wheeler, and A. Donabedian. Market-oriented cost-containment strategies and quality of care. *Milbank Mem. Fund Q.* 1982; 60:518–50.

61. Grossman, R.M. A review of physician cost-containment strategies for laboratory testing. *Med. Care.* 1983; 21:783–802.

62. Myers, L.P., and S.A. Schroeder. Physician use of services for the hospitalized patient: A review, with implications for cost containment. *Milbank Mem. Fund Q.* 1981; 59:481–507.

63. See references 54–62 above.

64. Abrams, H.L. The 'overutilization' of x-rays. *N. Engl. J. Med.* 1979; 300:1213–16.

65. Bloomgarden, Z., and V.W. Sidel. Evaluation of utilization of laboratory tests in a hospital emergency room. *Am. J. Public Health.* 1980; 70:525–28.

66. Hall, F.M. Overutilization of radiological examinations. *Radiology.* 1976; 120:443–48.

67. Eisenberg, J.M. An educational program to modify laboratory use by house staff. *J. Med. Educ.* 1977; 52:578–81.

68. Eisenberg, J.M. The use of ancillary services: A role for utilization review? *Med. Care.* 1982; 20:849–61.

69. Schroeder, S.A., L.P. Myers, and S.J. McPhee. The failure of physician education as a cost containment strategy: Report of a prospective controlled trial at a university hospital. *J.A.M.A.* 1984; 252:225–30.

70. Eisenberg, J.M., S.V. Williams, L. Garner, R. Viale, and H. Smits. Computer-based audit to detect and correct overutilization of laboratory tests. *Med. Care.* 1977; 15:915–21.

71. Collen, M.F. *Utilization of Diagnostic X-Ray Examinations.* Washington, D.C.: National Center for Devices and Radiological Health, Food and Drug Administration; Public Health Service; August 1983.

72. See reference 68 above.

73. Knapp, D.E., D.A. Knapp, M.K. Speedie, D.M. Yaeger, and C.L. Baker. Relationship of inappropriate drug prescribing to increased length of hospital stay. *Am. J. Hosp. Pharm.* 1979; 36:1334–37.

74. Maronde, R.F., P.V. Lee, M.M. McCarron, and S. Seibert. A study of prescribing patterns. *Med. Care.* 1971; 9:383–95.

75. Brook, R.H., K.N. Williams, and J.E. Rolph. Controlling the use and cost of medical services: The New Mexico Experimental Medical Care Review Organization—a four year case study. *Med. Care.* 1978; 16(suppl):1–76.

76. Ray, W.A., C.F. Federspiel, and W. Schaffner. Prescribing of tetracycline to children less than 8 years old. *J.A.M.A.* 1977; 237:2069–74.

77. Ray, W.A., C.F. Federspiel, and W. Schaffner. A study of antipsychotic drug use in nursing homes: Epidemiologic evidence suggesting misuse. *Am. J. Public Health.* 1980; 70:485–91.

78. Gertman, P.M., and J.D. Restuccia. The appropriateness evaluation protocol: A technique for assessing unnecessary days of hospital care. *Med. Care.* 1981; 19:855–71.

79. McCarthy, E.G., and M.L. Finkel. Second opinion elective surgery programs: Outcome status over time. *Med. Care.* 1978; 16:984–94.

80. Bailit, H.L., and J. Clive. The development of dental practice profiles. *Med. Care.* 1981; 19:30–46.

81. Vautrain, R.L., and P.F. Griner. Physician's orders, use of nursing resources, and subsequent clinical events. *J. Med. Educ.* 1978; 53:125–28.

82. See reference 24 above.

83. Bunker, J.P., H.S. Luft, and A. Enthoven. Should surgery be regionalized? *Surg. Clin. North Am.* 1982; 62:657–68.

84. Connell, F.A., L.A. Blide, and M.A. Hanken. Clinical correlates of small area variation in population based admission rates for diabetes. *Med. Care.* 1984; 22:939–49.

85. Lundberg, G.D. Perseveration of laboratory test ordering: A syndrome affecting clinicians. *J.A.M.A.* 1983; 249:639.

86. Williams, S.V., J.M. Eisenberg, L.A. Pascale, and D.S. Kitz. Physicians' perceptions about unnecessary diagnostic testing. *Inquiry.* 1982; 19:363–70.

87. See reference 50 above.

88. Roemer, M.I. Bed supply and hospital utilization: A natural experiment. *Hospitals.* 1961; 35:36–42.

89. See reference 25 above.

90. Cageorge, S.M., and L.L. Roos. When surgical rates change: Workload and turnover in Manitoba 1974–1978. *Med. Care.* 1984; 22:890–900.

91. See reference 90 above.

92. Singer, D.E., P.L. Carr, A.G. Mulley, and G.E. Thibault. Rationing intensive care—physician responses to a resource shortage. *N. Engl. J. Med.* 1983; 309:1155–60.

93. See reference 1 above.

94. See reference 18 above.

95. See reference 14 above.

96. Fuchs, V.R. *Who Shall Live? Health, Economics and Social Change.* New York: Basic Books, 1974.

97. See reference 13 above.

98. See reference 8 above.

99. See reference 9 above.

100. See reference 18 above.

101. Fuchs, V.R. The supply of surgeons and the demand for operations. *J. Hum. Resour.* 1978; 13(suppl):35–56.

102. Mitchell, J.B., and J. Cromwell. Variations in surgery rates and the supply of surgeons. In Rothberg, D.L., ed. *Regional Variations in Hospital Use.* Lexington, Mass.: Lexington Books, 1982; 103–30.

103. See reference 5 above.

104. See reference 50 above.

105. See reference 14 above.

106. See reference 1 above.

107. See reference 9 above.

108. Hornbrook, M.C., and M.G. Goldfarb. A partial test of a hospital behavioral model. *Soc. Sci. Med.* 1983; 17:667–80.

109. Munch, P. Economic incentives to order lab tests: Theory and evidence. In

Hough, D.E., and G.I. Misek, eds. *Socioeconomic Issues of Health.* Chicago: American Medical Assoc., 1980; 59–83.

110. See reference 18 above.

111. Rossiter, L.F., and G.R. Wilensky. A reexamination of the use of physician services: The role of physician-initiated demand. *Inquiry.* 1983; 20:162–72.

112. See reference 4 above.

113. See reference 3 above.

114. See reference 3 above.

115. Arrow, K.J. Uncertainty and the welfare economics of medical care. *Am. Econ. Rev.* 1963; 53:941–73.

116. Feldstein, M.S. The rising price of physicians' services. *Rev. Stat.* 1970; 52:121–33.

117. Evans, R.C. Supplier-induced demand: Some empirical evidence and implications. In Perlman, M., ed. *The Economics of Health and Medical Care.* New York: John Wiley & Sons, 1974; 1–547.

118. See reference 3 above.

119. See reference 111 above.

120. Rice, T.H. The impact of changing Medicare reimbursement rates on physician-induced demand. *Med. Care.* 1983; 21:803–15.

121. Roos, L.L., Jr. Supply, workload and utilization: A population-based analysis of surgery in rural Manitoba. *Am. J. Public Health.* 1983; 73:414–21.

122. See reference 120 above.

123. See reference 121 above.

124. Hemenway, D., and D. Fallon. Testing for physician-induced demand with hypothetical cases. *Med. Care.* 1985; 23:344–49.

125. See reference 3 above.

126. See reference 111 above.

127. Eisenberg, J.M., and J.C. Hershey. Derived thresholds: Determining the diagnostic probabilities at which clinicians initiate testing and treatment. *Med. Decis. Making.* 1983; 3:155–68.

128. Pauker, S.G., and J.P. Kassirer. The threshold approach to clinical decision making. *N. Engl. J. Med.* 1980; 302:1109–17.

129. See reference 127 above.

2

The Physician as
Self-Fulfilling Practitioner

One set of influences on medical decision making serves the physicians' own interests, including—but not limited to—the desire for income. This chapter addresses the ways in which physicians make decisions in their own interests. Subsequent chapters discuss other faces of the physician as decision maker: the doctor acting on behalf of the patient's interest and the doctor acting in the interest of society as a whole. Obviously, these roles may come into conflict in some decisions, such as when the expenditure of vast amounts of resources to prolong a patient's life by a few months may not be the most effective use of society's resources.

A component of the decision-making process will include some degree of economic self-interest as the physician decides whether to recommend medical services. However, many economic assessments of the physicians' role in medical care utilization have considered only the effect of their expected income on medical decision making. Even setting aside physicians' concern for their patients' well-being and preferences and their concern for the social good, this model of pure economic determinism of physician behavior is an oversimplification. "Self-fulfilling physicians," whose practices are motivated by self-interest, will seek to gain more from their actions than income alone. Self-interest is a more complex concept than simply the acquisition of money. The physicians will weigh, among other considerations, the time they will have for activities other than work, the style of practice they prefer, and the image to which they aspire in the community. Influencing these decisions will be the physicians' personal characteristics, the nature of the practice setting, and the influence of fellow professionals. The influences on medical decision making which satisfy personal desires of the physician as a self-fulfilling practitioner and which are discussed in this chapter include:

1. Desire for income
2. Desire for a style of practice
3. The physician's personal characteristics
4. The practice setting
5. Standards established by clinical leadership

Although this discussion emphasizes the utilization of existing medical services, its arguments are applicable to the diffusion of new services as well. The diffusion of medical innovations, described at length in the literature, can be considered a special case of medical care utilization. Whereas some factors may influence physicians' prescription of an already available service more or less than they affect the prescription of a new service, the sets of influences are convergent. In fact, some differences among physicians' utilization patterns that are shown in cross-sectional studies of utilization may simply be due to different groups of physicians being at different stages in the process of accepting or rejecting medical innovations.

The Physician as an Income Seeker

The notion that physicians are motivated by a desire for personal income has received careful attention by health economists. A rational person living in a society in which money is needed for basic necessities and luxuries (and in which money is a determinant of social status) would be expected to seek income, and economists have studied the nature and magnitude of income as an influence on medical practice patterns. Although some have suggested that physicians seek to maximize their income, most have proposed that physicians seek a target income or that they strike a balance between income and other desires such as leisure [1–3]. Additional income can be gained either by capturing some of society's unmet demand for medical care or by creating demand [4].

Some evidence for the influence that physicians' desire for income has on practice patterns derives from studies of the relationship between the supply of physicians and the cost and volume of medical practice. The literature on physician-induced demand implies that physicians can create demand to generate income, as described in chapter 1, but the effect of physician supply alone on utilization is generally agreed to be weak.

For example, Fuchs showed that a 10 percent increase in the surgeon-to-population ratio led to a modest 3 percent increase in the number of operations per capita [5]. However, in addition to the increase in per-capita surgical rates, the increase in the supply of surgeons was accompanied by an increase in fees charged for those operations. Therefore, despite a 7 percent decrease in the average surgeon's workload, the surgeons acted to protect their incomes by inducing more demand (shifting the demand curve), rather than providing more operations at a lower price (which would be expected if the supply had changed without a shift of the demand curve). The effect of surgical supply was greater on the cost of care than it was on utilization alone.

Although the theory of induced demand remains controversial and the degree to which physicians can create work for themselves to generate income is not well established, there is reasonable evidence that doctors do adjust the services they provide in response to economic incentives. Even if doctors do not induce new demand, they may substitute one of their services for another. Some economists have argued that doctors may substitute inpatient for outpatient visits or laboratory tests for time spent with the patient in the office, in order to keep the quality of care constant [6, 7]. Although the assumption that medical services can be easily substituted for one another without a change in quality is clinically naive, some substitution of this sort certainly does occur. Because doctors cannot instantly adjust the size or characteristics of their patient load, they may respond in different ways to the medical problems that their patients present. This argument suggests that, in the short run, doctors may treat their patients' complaints in a way that is influenced by financial considerations, while in the long run they may also attempt to change their patient load to bring their hours and income back into equilibrium [7].

Some of the most convincing evidence that physicians' opportunity for income affects their practice patterns is available from studies of situations in which physicians' fees were reduced. These natural experiments demonstrate how doctors change their practices in response to financial incentives. They may change the volume of services they provide, alter the mix of services, change the way in which the services are labeled, or change the site at which medical care is delivered to the patient.

In California, when prices were frozen during the Economic Stabilization Program in 1971, physicians increased the number of services provided to Medicare recipients and altered their mix so that higher billings resulted [8, 9]. Large increases were seen in the provision of almost all types of physician services, including office and hospital visits as well as ancillary services such as radiographic examinations, laboratory tests, and electrocardiograms. When the price controls were lifted in 1975, physicians raised their prices by 23 percent and the quantity of services declined (by 9 percent for general practitioners). Gabel and Rice have pointed out that Medicare claims in this California study could not show whether the increases in the quantity and intensity of services were actual (thereby suggesting that the doctors had, in fact, induced demand) or whether the increased billings simply reflected changes in physicians' billing practices [10]. For example, doctors might have unbundled their services, billing separately for laboratory tests that were formerly included as part of the office visit fee. Physicians also may have relabeled their charges so that an office visit would be described as being more intense, such as renaming a "brief" visit as "intermediate." Similar results were found for Medicaid services provided by physicians during the period that payments were frozen. In fact, when payment levels rose in 1976, physicians decreased the complexity of services billed to Medicaid by 2 percent to 6 percent. Therefore, although the California payment freeze was successful in holding down prices, it was ineffective in modifying physicians' total revenue.

A second natural experiment illustrated a similar response to a change in physicians' fees. A 30 percent reduction in fees for surgery by Medicaid in Massachusetts led to a decrease in the number of physicians participating in Medicaid and, for some surgery in some areas, an increase in the number of operations per participating physician. Overall, surgical utilization increased; only tonsillectomies and adenoidectomies showed a strong indication of a decline in the level of surgery after the fee cut [11].

In a third natural experiment, when Medicare payment schedules in Colorado were revised, changes in the volume of services occurred to maintain physicians' income [12]. Rice found that declining reimbursement rates resulted in the provision of more intensive services, but that for those physicians whose Medicare reimbursement rates increased, the intensity of services provided decreased. A 1 percent decrease in the reimbursement rate resulted in a 0.61 percent increase in intensity of medical service. The elasticity of surgical services was substantially less; a 1 percent decline in the surgical reimbursement rate resulted in an increase of 0.15 percent in the intensity of surgical service provided. The elasticity for laboratory tests was such that a 1 percent decrease in reimbursement for tests would result in a 0.52 percent increase in services provided. No evidence was seen of demand inducement for radiology services. Surprisingly, there was no apparent relationship between the reimbursement rate for office visits and the resulting number of laboratory tests ordered. Therefore, doctors' responses to the Colorado changes in reimbursement, with some fees increasing and some decreasing, provide strong evidence that physicians do alter the volume and type of services they provide in response to changes in the price of those services.

In the five years after Quebec introduced its universal health insurance system in 1970, the fees paid to physicians were not increased. In response, Quebec physicians increased the reported complexity of the services they provided, according to research conducted by Berry [13]. In 1971, "ordinary" examinations comprised 88 percent of all examinations provided by physicians, but by 1975 "ordinary" examinations had declined to 60 percent. Conversely, "comprehensive" examinations increased from 1 percent to 5 percent of the total. Over the five-year period, general practitioners provided 19 percent fewer office visits, but revenue per visit increased by 19 percent. Gabel and Rice, writing about strategies to reduce public expenditures for physician services, have described this situation as the "price of paying less"—that is, freezing fees alone is not an effective method for controlling overall costs [14].

Other evidence for the effect of expected income on physician utilization patterns is provided by Fuchs and Kramer, who concluded that higher prices do not induce the provision of additional services from physicians [15]. Consistent with the research on the effect of changes in fees, they suggested that the opposite may occur—that higher prices are accompanied by a decrease in the number of services supplied. These findings suggest that physicians may not operate as a profit-maximizing firm would be expected to behave according to traditional microeconomic theory (by increasing volume of services provided in response to an increase in the price). Similarly, Brook and colleagues found that constraints on the use of certain injectable drugs led physicians to replace use of these drugs with other services for which they could bill, presumably to maintain their levels of income [16, 17].

Some of the most extensive research on doctors' responses to financial incentives was carried out in conjunction with the multimillion-dollar Rand Health Insurance Experiment [18–21]. Analysis of surveys on physician practice costs and incomes and data from the Rand experiment suggest that physicians will substitute laboratory tests for time spent with patients if third-party allowable charges for office visits are reduced. In contrast to the the Colorado case [22], the Rand group studied a 1975 situation in which controls on office visit fees were at least partially offset by higher fees for laboratory tests [23, 24]. If reimbursement for tests is not constrained and charges for the physicians' time are limited, the researchers conclude, the physician will vary test prices to achieve the optimal total price for the visit. However, with today's controls on prices of laboratory tests, doctors may not have as much leeway as they did earlier in adjusting their charges for these tests. Therefore, doctors today might be more likely to respond by increasing the volume rather than the price of ancillary services.

Fee-for-service medicine, in which physicians are paid on the basis of the volume of services they provide, has been blamed for overutilization of services because it yields incentives for overprovision. For example, length of stay, consultation rates, and the use of ancillary services seem to be lower when physicians are compensated on a salaried basis than when they are paid fee for service [25].

An interesting experiment in physician reimbursement has shed light on the role of fee-for-service practice in utilization by physicians. In 1975 and 1976, Pennsylvania Blue Shield enrolled 91 physicians practicing in nine hospitals throughout the State in an experimental plan [26]. The doctors agreed to accept payment by case for hospitalized patients, rather than by visit to the patient. Hospitals were paid in the traditional per-diem manner. This voluntary experimental program established per-case fees for 24 disease classifications. In four of the seven hospitals with enough data to be analyzed, the average length of stay for these patients decreased. Overall, length of stay showed a small (3 percent) but statistically significant decrease. Per-case reimbursement was most effective in reducing length of stay at hospitals with lower occupancy rates. Markel concluded that this result suggests hospitals with low occupancy rates may seek to maintain higher occupancy by tolerating some slack in their lengths of stay. Per-case reimbursement may have been effective primarily in reducing this slack, since the physicians were given an inducement to decrease length of stay. Interestingly, the Pennsylvania Blue Shield experiment resulted in higher levels of payment to doctors but lower rates to the hospitals. The increased Blue Shield payment to physicians was more than compensated for by reduced Blue Cross payments to the hospital.

Although these results suggest that fee-for-service payment of physicians induces greater costs by rewarding higher volumes of service with higher revenue, Pauly has suggested that this is not necessarily the case [27]. He has proposed that it is not the fee-for-service system that induces overprovision, but rather the level of existing fees for some procedures.

A case in point may be the fee structure for ancillary services compared with that for office visits to primary care practitioners. Even conservative estimates reveal the average profits for different tests in office practice to vary sixfold, ranging from about six dollars for an electrocardiogram to about one dollar for a urinalysis [28, 29]. An internist can triple his income by providing and charging for a simple battery of diagnostic tests, such as radiologic, laboratory, and electrocardiographic procedures [30]. Figure 2.1 illustrates these large differences in net income that depend on whether the physician performs and bills for a variety of tests. This simulation, developed by Schroeder and Showstack in the mid-1970s, shows the charges and net income that a solo practitioner could expect with four different types of practice arrangements for diagnostic testing. Model A represents an office in which no procedures or tests are done. Model B is an office in which five basic procedures and tests are done (electrocardiography, urinalysis, complete blood count, sigmoidoscopy, and tuberculin skin test), as is Model C, but in Model C a

Figure 2.1   Four models of financial incentives to perform medical procedures and laboratory tests in solo office practice showing annual gross charges, expenses, noncollectables, and net income for each practice model.

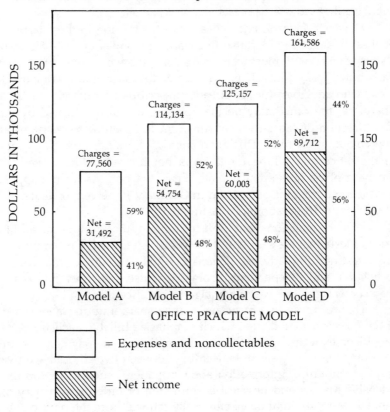

Source: Schroeder and Showstack [29]. Reprinted by permission of *Medical Care*, 1978; 16:295.

higher proportion of patients receive these tests. Model D is an office in which three additional tests are performed (chest radiography, cardiovascular treadmill stress test, and automated 12-channel blood chemistry test).

Whether a physician has the equipment to perform diagnostic tests in the office may be an important determinant of the ancillary services prescribed. In fact, ownership of radiographic equipment by the prescribing physician has been shown to be the most important influence on radiology use, which is two-thirds higher than the rates for comparable physicians who do not own their own equipment [31]. Furthermore, physicians who purchase diagnostic tests and then bill their patients, do more tests than physicians who refer patients to laboratories that directly bill the patient [32]. Bailey has suggested that this potential for profit in laboratory testing for physicians who perform tests in their offices encourages them to overuse tests [33].

However, Danzon and colleagues urge caution in the interpretation of these results [34]. Because there are economies of scale for in-office testing (that is, with more tests being done, the average cost of performing each test is less), physicians who decide to test in-house are likely to be those who anticipate (or are already prescribing) a high volume of tests. Therefore, the cause may be the opposite of that postulated by Bailey. The direction of causality may run from test volume to decisions about how to obtain the tests. This phenomenon of providing ancillary services in the office and billing for them is not limited to the United States. Japanese physicians often operate their own pharmacies to supplement their income from office fees and in Germany 15 percent of all income for physicians is from laboratory testing [35].

Recent regulations that limit the amount that doctors can add to the price of tests that are sent out of the office, offer further incentives for in-office testing. Similarly, regulations for quality assurance that apply only to hospital and independent laboratories raise their operating costs and may confer a relative cost advantage to in-office testing [36].

This response by physicians to the usual reimbursement schedules of fee-for-service medicine, which emphasize billable ancillary services, should be expected given the values implicit in the payment schedules. For example, if a physician is deciding between two clinically equivalent ways of obtaining information about a patient, such as performing an extensive history and physical examination or ordering a battery of diagnostic tests, it might be economically rational from the physician's perspective to order the tests. Because hospital and ancillary services are generally more handsomely reimbursed by third-party payers, the physicians may substitute these services for their own time, even if doing so is not efficient for the system. Pauly has argued that this substitution would be efficient for physicians (and sometimes for patients) [37]. Physicians would be responding appropriately to the incentives that are offered to them by the medical care system if they were to refer the patients to consultants, hospitalize the patients, or order laboratory tests or radiologic examinations. Furthermore, minimizing the overall costs of medical care may be counter to the physicians' personal economic interests if doing so takes time to learn.

Pauly also suggests that physicians' ability to manipulate demand to provide personal income is dependent on their ability to manipulate their patients' knowledge of the marginal utility of additional care (that is, the potential contribution of medical services to their health). Although physicians probably do not purposely or maliciously manipulate the accuracy of the information they provide to patients in order to induce demand (particularly since they may not have accurate information themselves), Pauly's argument does emphasize the usually uninformed state of medical care consumers and their dependence on their providers for advice about the services they should receive.

Of course, physicians may not always manipulate demand to increase the number of services for which they can bill, even if this practice is in their short-run financial interests. Other factors that are reviewed in this and the next two chapters may constrain the physician from prescribing profitable but clinically marginal services. Even in the absence of nonfinancial incentives that constrain the prescription of services, physicians may realize that their short-term economic benefit could be at the cost of lost income in the future. For example, if patients (or third-party payers) are charged substantially higher costs for medical care, they might go to other physicians (or other organizations, such as health maintenance organizations) to seek lower medical costs. In this era of increasing competition, of changing systems of health care delivery, and of increased cost consciousness by those paying for medical care, these long-term economic perspectives may play an increasingly important role in medical decision making.

On the other hand, other forces such as decreased marginal income tax rates and the impending oversupply of physicians may cause doctors to be more willing to induce demand for their services. This inducement could take place in the traditional fashion, with the individual doctor advising the patient that more medical care services are recommended, but inducement may well take new forms such as advertising or the creation of new services for potential but previously unmet demand (for example, wellness care).

Style of Practice

In addition to seeking personal income, physicians are motivated by the style of medicine that they desire to practice and the lifestyle that they seek outside practice. Although physicians' leisure time is considered in the economic model that suggests a tradeoff between labor and leisure, other elements of their personal style and preferences have received less attention.

Wennberg and Gittelsohn have described the presence of different styles of practice among surgeons, which they describe as "surgical signatures" [38]. Differences in both the rates and types of surgery are due, in part, to differences in practice styles among practitioners [39, 40]. Whereas physicians may have originally adopted these styles of practice for clinical or economic reasons, they often become entrenched in habit [41]. Habit was perceived by community practitioners in one survey to be an important cause of overuse of diagnostic tests [42]. Physicians' attitudes and values have been shown to play an important role in the decision to admit infants to a neonatal intensive care unit [43]. Different styles of practice in the hospital have also been shown to result in different demands for nursing time [44].

Roos has suggested that "hysterectomy-prone" primary care physicians are most likely to be gynecologists or general practitioners, even when patients are excluded who were likely to have been referred for this reason [45]. These hysterectomy-prone physicians were more likely to perform the surgery than other doctors. These findings suggest that doctors' practice styles may be influenced, at least in part, by economic motivation, although the surgeon's characteristic desire to operate may transcend financial rewards.

Several investigators have shown that personality traits of the physician may also affect utilization patterns [46–48]. Physicians who are early adopters of innovations tend to be cosmopolitan and ideologically liberal physicians.

The characteristics of the patients whom physicians want to have in their practices also affect medical decision making. Physicians whose practices are busy and who must turn away patients often use discretion in doing so. For example, gynecologists often choose not to retain patients complaining of obesity, but to refer them to endocrinologists instead [49]. Doctors who seek a certain style of practice may encourage or discourage follow-up visits, referrals, and even first visits on the basis of a patient's race, sex, age, or social status [50]. Although these characteristics of patients are usually thought to govern medical care utilization because of their effect on patient-initiated demand, they also seem to affect demand induced by physicians who are seeking a certain style of practice or who respond differently to different types of patients.

Physicians prefer to care for certain types of clinical problems as well as certain types of patients. The desire of gynecologists to refer obese patients may be due to the patient's appearance, but it may also be due to the gynecologist's desire to see "interesting patients." Desirable patients are often those who have unusual or challenging medical problems and those for whom diagnosis and therapy are likely to lead to gratifying, successful outcomes. Physicians' desires for a certain style of practice may result from their personal values or from the social or personal satisfaction that they place on caring for different types of patients. However, this kind of discretion in the selection of patients may be possible only when physicians can "afford" not to accept patients. This situation occurs when the payment for medical care is equal to the cost to the physicians of seeing the patients (including the opportunity cost of their own time—a measure of how they could spend their time otherwise) at a quantity of care that is less than that demanded from them. This suggests that it would not be worth it to the physicians to see more patients at this price or at a lower price that might have to be offered in order to attract them. The demand for care at this price is greater than the supply physicians want to make available at the price. At this point, the physicians can choose the patients they will treat [51]. Obviously, if physicians can create this excess demand, they will be able to ensure themselves discretion in the choice of patients.

Convenience of the physician may play a role in some utilization decisions as well, but the confounding influence of opportunity costs (how doctors would use the time otherwise) makes these behaviors difficult to interpret. For example, Kaiser-Permanente physicians whose offices are located at hospitals admit 44 percent more patients and use 44 more hospital days per 1000 outpatient visits than do Kaiser physicians whose offices are elsewhere [52, 53]. That the lengths of stay, numbers of laboratory tests, and numbers of consultations of these physicians are less than those of physicians who are not hospital based could reflect greater efficiency but could also reflect the admission of patients who are less ill. Fee-for-service doctors also seem to be influenced by their own convenience in their decisions to hospitalize patients. This reason may explain why, in one study, solo practitioners (who do not have coverage that is as easily shared as group practice members) and physicians with busy outpatient practices were less likely to hospitalize patients when clinical variables were controlled [54]. Convenience also helps to explain why physician staffing shortages in hospitals coincide with increased referrals of infants to neonatal intensive care units [55] and why the peak periods of the day for ordering stat tests are just before the times when rounds are made (for which test results are needed) or when physicians are about to leave in the evening [56]. It cannot be denied that quality of care may play a role in these decisions to transfer patients to an intensive care unit or to request immediate turnaround on diagnostic tests, but these findings do suggest that certain physician practices are driven by a desire for convenience.

Physicians' Characteristics

Along with physicians' desires for income and certain styles of practice, physicians' own personal characteristics affect their practice patterns. These characteristics include specialty, age, sex, experience, and type of training. Some characteristics, such as age and experience, are obviously beyond the control of the physician and cannot be changed at will. Others are relatively fixed once the initial decision has been made; for example, although specialty and type of training can be changed in midcareer, it is unusual to do so. Therefore, these personal characteristics of the individual physician are relatively fixed and represent a sort of "physician portrait." Characteristic practice patterns typify these portraits and help to explain interphysician variation [57].

Specialization has received the most attention for its influence on physician behavior. In general, the literature suggests that more specialized physicians provide more intensive care than do generalists. For example, general practitioners (but not necessarily those who are family physicians) order fewer diagnostic tests than do internists [58–60]. Similarly, pediatricians order significantly more diagnostic tests for common childhood illnesses than general practitioners do [61]. When attending physicians are responsible for test ordering at a teaching hospital, subspecialists order more tests than general internists [62]. These differences in test ordering among physicians in different specialties are apparent as early as residency [63]. There is evidence that residents learn these different decision-making styles in the course of their residency training [64]. Although some differences in decision-making style may reflect the choice of a specialty with which individuals believe they will be comfortable, clearly a substantial amount of socialization and establishment of practice style occurs during the residency.

For example, at one teaching hospital, housestaff in medicine, neurology, and pediatrics had markedly different use rates of tuberculosis cultures when they examined cerebrospinal fluid [65]. Whereas only 6 percent of the cerebrospinal specimens were cultured for tuberculosis by pediatric residents, 65 percent and 71 percent were cultured by medicine and neurology residents, respectively. These practices persisted despite the low actual probability of tuberculous meningitis in all but a few patients on the three services. The investigators who identified these differences suggest that informal clinical policies had developed within these communities of physicians and had persisted over six years despite changes in the composition of the resident groups each year.

These differences in the ordering of diagnostic tests have been interpreted as reflecting different levels of intensity of care by different types of specialists. A difference in style of practice has also been seen in the amount of time spent by physicians with their patients during office visits, with internists spending more time per patient than family physicians and general practitioners [66].

The differences in the intensity of care by different specialists would be expected (and probably desirable) if more specialized physicians cared for patients who are more severely ill. However, in studies in which case mix and severity of illness have been controlled as well as possible, these differences have often remained. The study by Eisenberg and Nicklin is one exception; there, differences in the rates of utilization of laboratory tests and radiologic examinations between family physicians and internists disappeared when case mix and severity of illness were taken into account [67]. Even so, both family physicians and internists provided more intensive care than did general practitioners.

Because most studies have not been able to separate the practice patterns of family physicians and general practitioners, these two specialties have unfortunately been merged in many analyses of utilization. When the utilization data of these two groups are merged, it becomes impossible to determine whether the two groups of physicians practice in a similar manner. The results of the study by Eisenberg and Nicklin suggest that family physicians, with their three-year residencies, board certification, and continuing education requirements, may practice more like internists than like general practitioners [68].

The problem of discerning differences in case mix can make it difficult to evaluate variation among physicians in surgical rates, as well as in rates of ancillary services such as laboratory tests. By selecting subpopulations that eliminated women referred to gynecologists and surgeons for surgery in Manitoba, Roos demonstrated that certain types of physicians are "hysterectomy-prone" [69]. Of physicians serving as primary care physicians in Manitoba, 44 percent of gynecologists, 4 percent of general practitioners, 9 percent of general surgeons, and 3 percent of internists were especially likely to have primary care patients in their practices undergo a hysterectomy. Because of the larger number of general practitioners than general surgeons, a larger proportion of hysterectomy-prone doctors were general practitioners.

Using the same claims data from Manitoba, Roos and colleagues studied physicians' hospitalization practices and demonstrated that even the limited clinical information from claims can help to control for differences in case mix [70]. When patients are classified by characteristics such as the primary diagnoses on hospitalization, the number of different diagnoses on ambulatory visits, deaths and admission to nursing homes within three years, and age, systematic differences among physicians' use of hospital beds could be demonstrated. For example, rural physicians, younger physicians, and those trained outside Canada and Britain averaged more hospital days per patient in their primary care panels. When case mix was controlled, physicians with appointments at teaching hospitals averaged fewer hospital days per primary patient. Whether rural physicians, who practice at hospitals that have lower occupany rates, admit and readmit their patients more often because of the availability of beds or because of the difficulty patients might have with outpatient care in more isolated rural areas could not be answered by this study. Nonetheless, the study was important in its demonstration that wide variation in physicians' admission and readmission rates, as well as length of stay, does persist after controlling for case mix as well as can be done with claims data.

Another way to control for case-mix differences among physicians is to ask them to respond to clinical vignettes. One such study found no difference in test ordering among doctors of different specialties, but all of the doctors studied were at a university medical center [71]. This homogeneity, the use of only two vignettes, and the small sample size (no power analysis was done to determine whether important differences were likely to have been missed) means that this study could have underestimated interspecialty differences in test use.

Reasons other than the intensity of care may explain differences in utilization among specialists. For example, the finding that gynecologists more often refer patients to endocrinologists to evaluate obesity than do internists and family practitioners suggests that gynecologists have a more limited area of focus than do generalist physicians [72].

Few studies have failed to show a difference in utilization among the specialties, but there have been exceptions. Dietrich and Goldberg found no difference in the preventive services provided by different types of specialists [73]. Even if many of the apparent differences among the specialties are due to unmeasured differences in case mix and severity of illness, evidence is still convincing that some differences do persist.

Whereas the physician's sex seems to have no measurable effect on practice style [74, 75], age is related to levels of utilization. In general, younger physicians prescribe more services. These results have been demonstrated repeatedly [76 –80] and with few exceptions [81, 82]. Figures 2.2 and 2.3 show the results of a study of diagnostic test use by doctors of different ages [83], demonstrating lower use by older physicians, both for x-ray and laboratory tests. One study that did not show higher test use by younger doctors involved only 30 internists and used a cut-off point of 20 years since graduation from medical school to define younger and older doctors, thereby potentially overlooking changes at younger ages [84].

The generally higher levels of utilization by younger physicians could occur because they have not yet had time to mature clinically, to understand the limitations of testing, and to gain experience in clinical judgement. These findings would imply overutilization by younger doctors. On the other hand, these age-related differences could also be explained by a lack of knowledge and familiarity among the older clinicians with recently developed diagnostic tests. This argument would imply underutilization by the older physicians. Evidence indicates that both reasons are true.

Figure 2.2   Older doctors use fewer laboratory tests.

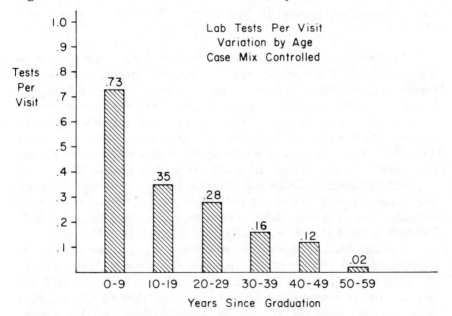

Source: Eisenberg and Nicklin [65]. Reprinted by permission of *Medical Care*, 1981; 19:304.

Figure 2.3   Older doctors use fewer radiologic tests.

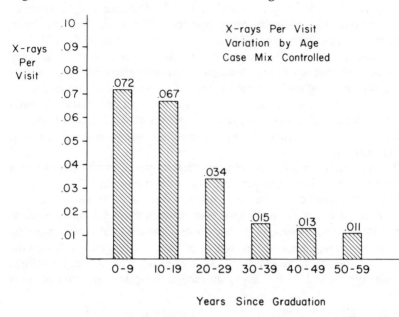

Source: Eisenberg and Nicklin [65]. Reprinted by permission of *Medical Care*, 1981; 19:305.

The larger number of tests that are ordered by younger physicians is accompanied by shorter lengths of stay [85, 86]. This more intense and perhaps more efficient style of practice may reflect the leading edge of changes in medical care. Because teaching hospitals' practices are particularly influenced by the styles of younger doctors, this finding would help to explain why teaching hospitals tend to have larger numbers of tests per admission but shorter lengths of stay. Innovations also are adopted more often by younger, more technically competent doctors [87].

Although this evidence suggests that younger doctors order more tests because they are more clinically sophisticated, physicians seem to decrease their use of medical services as they gain clinical maturity [88]. Residents order slightly more tests than do faculty [89] and when attending physicians become responsible for ordering diagnostic tests at a teaching hospital, they order 20 percent fewer tests than the residents had [90]. These differences in test ordering are seen within the years of residency as well. First-year residents have higher bills for laboratory testing than do more senior residents [91, 92]. The American Board of Internal Medicine has found that the number of diagnostic tests ordered by physicians taking its pilot computer-based examination of simulated cases is inversely related to the individual's level of training [93]. The same improvement has been shown for the prescription of tranquilizers, which is appropriately lower among more experienced clinicians [94].

Although the clinical maturity of clinicians does seem to be related to the greater appropriateness and lower volume of services prescribed, evidence on the influence of the type of training is less clear. Physicians who have been educated at schools and hospitals with scientific medical orientations generally use fewer resources when the case is relatively unambiguous, but use more when ambiquity is high [95]. In contrast, another study found that physicians trained in medical schools with academic orientations ordered more tests for hypertensive patients, but that ambiguity was not related to test use [96]. Still another study suggested that graduates of prestigious schools order fewer services [97].

The results of studies on the utilization rates by foreign medical graduates are also conflicting. Although some evidence shows that foreign medical graduates prescribe fewer services [98], studies in which case mix is controlled show foreign graduates to use more diagnostic tests [99].

Most investigators have found that specialty board certification is not related to levels of utilization [100–104]. However, the American Board of Internal Medicine has reported that candidates for certification who score better on the multiple-choice questions of knowledge also choose fewer diagnostic tests on the patient-management problems [105].

Therefore, it is clear that personal characteristics of physicians do influence their utilization of medical services, although some of the evidence is conflicting. Perhaps this discrepancy is due to the interaction of several characteristics of the doctors, such as financial and clinical factors. These numerous personal factors, including age, clinical experience, specialty, and type of education, do help to explain why variation in utilization among physicians exists even when the clinical situation is similar.

Practice Setting

In addition to economic factors, aspirations for a certain style of practice, and personal characteristics, the place where the physician practices also has an important influence on the level of utilization. Although many researchers who have reported variation among practice sites (such as different hospitals) have emphasized static descriptors such as bed supply, case mix, physician supply, or demographic characteristics of the service area [106], much of the interinstitutional variation in service utilization appears to be due to the interaction among professionals at the practice site.

The hospital has been described as a doctor's workshop that functions as a cooperative of physicians without effective, unified decision making [107, 108]. Despite the absence of centralized clinical decision making, hospitals clearly have practice styles. For physicians whom Friedson describes as "colleague-dependent," or desirous of approval by their peers, the influence of fellow professionals is particularly strong and produces a sort of group practice style [109].

Substantial evidence exists for the strong effect of peer pressure, professional leadership, and group styles of practice in determining the levels of use of various services [110–112]. These powerful effects of group style and clinical leadership are probably stronger in more formally organized practices. For example, physicians in a teaching hospital perceive pressure from others to be a major factor influencing the use of diagnostic tests [113]. This pressure seems to be translated into higher costs on teaching services, particularly for diagnostic testing [114, 115]. Although many have called for educational programs to offset this inflationary influence, wholesale reduction of teaching hospital services could adversely affect care if this reduction were done without regard to case mix or the necessity of services being provided. In fact, evidence from Stanford University Hospital suggests that the higher costs of treating patients on the faculty service were associated with decreased short-term mortality [116]. Whether long-term benefits actually result and whether the magnitude of benefit justifies the increased cost remain to be demonstrated. Nonetheless, it is clear that teaching services usually incur higher costs, at least in part because of a group ethos about the desired style of practice. The same kind of group ethos may also explain why doctors who practice in hospitals with lower occupancy rates are more likely to hospitalize their patients [117]. Apparently, physicians adjust their threshold for admission in accordance with the hospital's needs for inpatients.

Although health maintenance organizations (HMO) do have different financial incentives than fee-for-service practices, the organization of the HMO, rather than its financial structure, may be responsible for the lower rates of surgery and hospitalization seen with these organizations [118–120]. The lower rates of diagnostic test use by cardiologists practicing in HMO programs is due, in part, to differences among HMO and other cardiologists in their attitudes about coronary angiography and bypass surgery [121]. On the other hand, rheumatologists seem to provide equally intensive care to patients when case mix is carefully controlled [122]; and when fee-for-service patients do not have to pay coinsurance, the prescription of laboratory tests for these patients is not different from that for patients in prepaid practices [123]. Most savings in prepaid practices appear to occur because of savings in inpatient expenditures, probably for admissions of marginal necessity.

Several investigators have found a substantial intragroup cohesion among doctors who practice together in HMO groups. Whereas differences are often apparent among groups of HMO doctors, a practice style is usually shared by colleagues within the HMO [124]. At the Harvard Community Health Plan and other prepaid group practices [125], the role of peer pressure has been observed to be a key factor in determining utilization patterns, such as in the prescription of drugs [126, 127].

Pineault has suggested that this professional regulation in organized groups of physicians who practice together in collaboration is more important than the professional socialization that occurs during medical training [128]. The powerful influence of these group norms may explain why the prepaid group practice form of the HMO generally has lower utilization levels than individual practice associations, and why tightly organized fee-for-service group practices have levels of utilization that approach those of prepaid groups. This effect of peer pressure and influence, as well as the development of a group norm, may also explain why practitioners in larger group practices order, independent of patient characteristics, more diagnostic tests than doctors in smaller practices [129]. With larger groups, the pressure to conform to group standards may diffuse. The influence of the social climate among peers has also been observed to influence practice patterns in the United Kingdom [130].

Group norms of practice may extend beyond the informal influence of peer pressure. Eddy has described how group styles of practice may be translated into formal practice policy, but the establishment of practice rules or protocols can risk entrenching traditional practice and oversimplifying the complexities of clinical practice [131].

Obviously not all differences among practice sites can be explained by differences in the relationships of the practitioners and social norms. For example, teaching hospitals may perform more ancillary services simply because they usually have access to more advanced technology [132]. As others have pointed out, this higher volume of ancillary services in teaching hospitals may be partially balanced by decreased lengths of stay and may simply reflect the cutting edge of technical advancement—a universal trend toward shorter stays and more intensive treatment per day. Instead of representing fundamental differences among hospitals in their practice styles, the peculiar characteristics of teaching hospitals may reflect what is in store for other hospitals once the process of technological diffusion takes place [133, 134]. The increased use of services by urban hospitals may represent the same phenomenon of hospitals at different stages of adoption of technological innovations [135]; so might the shorter length of stay in West Coast hospitals reflect this phenomenon. The inability to discriminate whether interhospital differences are due to different degrees of practice evolution among hospitals may be an inevitable limitation of cross-sectional studies.

Despite the appeal of this argument that differences in utilization simply represent differing degrees of adoption of an inevitable technology or practice style, it cannot be denied that other real differences exist. For example, substantial variation in antenatal testing between clinic settings persists over time and involves both old and new technologies [136].

The Role of Clinical Leadership

One reason that different practice sites have different levels of utilization is the strong influence of their professional leadership. Certain physicians in every practice organization, be it a hospital or clinic practice, seem to be particularly influential in determining group norms of practice style. These individuals are often described as "educational influentials" because of their role as educators of the other staff about the practice of medicine [137, 138]. These influential physicians may not be members of the official hospital hierarchy, and doctors who are administratively influential may not be clinically influential. Although department chairmen and medical staff directors may often be influential clinically as well as administratively, often two independent hierarchies—clinical and administrative—exist, particularly in larger organizations.

The influence of clinical leadership has been clearly demonstrated in setting patterns of surgery [139, 140], in hospitalization rates and length of stay [141], in the use of diagnostic tests [142], and in drug prescribing [143–146]. Pharmaceutical manufacturers have long recognized the critical role of educationally influential doctors in the use of drugs, and they have targeted much of their marketing at the clinical leadership, in hopes of an eventual impact on the practice patterns of the leaders' colleagues.

The literature of health services research shows that the influence of professional leadership has been particularly prominent in physicians' acceptance of innovations [147, 148]. For example, the acceptance of computers in clinical practice is dependent on their adoption by leaders of professional networks [149]. The classic study of health care marketing by Coleman, Katz, and Menzel demonstrated the critical role of medical leadership in the prescription of a new drug [150]. In fact, most of the original research about the influence of clinical leadership on practice patterns has dealt with the adoption of innovations. Although several stages have been proposed in the process of adoption, investigators have found that the most crucial distinction is between first awareness and the decision to use an innovation. The medical literature is an important source of information, but professional colleagues are particularly influential in the final decision to change a medical practice. This process often occurs most effectively through informal channels, and the most potent legitimizing force for influencing medical practice is professional, face-to-face contact [151]. This contact operates on the general principles of diffusion networks [152]. Because so much information comes to physicians from commercial sources, some researchers have suggested that professional leaders have much to learn from the communication techniques of commercial concerns [153].

In summary, many of the factors that influence medical decision making do so because of the importance of the physician's personal desires and characteristics, as well as the professional influences on his behavior. Physicians, in attempting to satisfy their personal needs, will consider these important influences—whether consciously or unconsiously—as they prescribe medical services. A substantial portion of the well-documented variation in practice patterns is due to these effects of the physicians' desire for income and a certain style of practice, as well as to the influences of personal characteristics, the practice setting, and the clinical leadership.

References

1. Pauly, M.V. *Doctors and Their Workshops*. Chicago: National Bureau of Economic Research, The University of Chicago Press, 1980.

2. Sloan, F., J. Mitchell, and J. Cromwell. Physician participation in state Medicaid programs. *J. Hum. Resour.* 1978; 13(suppl):211–45.

3. Newhouse, J.P., W.G. Manning, C.N. Morris, et al. Some interim results from a controlled trial of cost sharing in health insurance. *N. Engl. J. Med.* 1981; 305:1501–7.

4. See reference 1 above.

5. Fuchs, V.R. The supply of surgeons and the demand for operations. *J. Hum. Resour.* 1978; 13(suppl):35–56.

6. McCombs, J.S. Physician treatment decisions in a multiple treatment model: The effects of physician supply. *J. Health Econ.* 1984; 3:155–71.

7. Feldman, R., R. Goldfarb, J. Rafferty, and M. Goldfarb. Physician choice of patient load and mode of treatment. *Atl. Econ. J.* 1981; 9:69–78.

8. Hadley, J. Physician participation in Medicaid: Evidence from California. *Health Serv. Res.* 1979; 14:266–80.

9. Gabel, J.R., and T.H. Rice. Reducing public expenditures for physician services: The price of paying less. *J. Health Polit. Policy Law.* 1985; 9:595–609.

10. See reference 9 above.

11. Schwartz, M., S.G. Martin, D.D. Cooper, G.M. Ljung, B.J. Whalen, and J. Blackburn. The effect of a thirty percent reduction in physician fees on Medicaid surgery rates in Massachusetts. *Am. J. Public Health.* 1981; 71:370–75.

12. Rice, T.H. The impact of changing Medicare reimbursement rates on physician-induced demand. *Med. Care.* 1983; 21:803–15.

13. Berry, C., P.J. Held, B. Kehrer, L. Marheim, and U. Reinhardt. Canadian physicians' supply response to Universal Health Insurance: The first years in Quebec (preliminary results). In Gabel, J.R., J. Taylor, N.T. Greenspan, and M. Blaxall, eds. *Physicians and Financial Incentives.* Washington, D.C.: U.S. Government Printing Office, 1980; 57–59.

14. See reference 9 above.

15. Fuchs, V.R., and M.J. Kramer. *Determinants of Expenditures for Physicians' Services in the United States 1948–68.* Washington, D.C.: National Center for Health Services Research and Development, Department of Health, Education and Welfare, December 1972; 1–63. DHEW publication no. (HSM) 73–3013.

16. Brook, R.H., K.N. Williams, and J.E. Rolph. Controlling the use and cost of medical services: The New Mexico Experimental Medical Care Review Organization—a four year case study. *Med. Care.* 1978; 16(suppl):1–76.

17. Brook, R.H., K.N. Williams, and J.E. Rolph. Use, costs, and quality of medical services: Impact of the New Mexico Peer Review System: A 1971–1975 study. *Ann. Intern. Med.* 1978; 89:256–63.

18. Danzon, P.M., W.G. Manning, and M.S. Marquis. Factors influencing laboratory test use and prices. *Health Care Financing Rev.* 1984; 5:23–32.

19. Danzon, P.M., W.G. Manning, and M.S. Marquis. *Factors Affecting Laboratory Test Use and Price.* Santa Monica, Calif.: Rand Corp., January 1983. Rand Corp. Pub. R–2987–HCFA.

20. Danzon, P.M. *Economic Factors in the Use of Laboratory Tests by Office-Based Physicians.* Santa Monica, Calif.: Rand Corp., August 1982. Rand Corp. Pub. R–2525–1–HCFA.

21. Marquis, M.S. *Laboratory Test Ordering by Physicians: The Effect of Reimbursement Policies.* Santa Monica, Calif.: Rand Corp., August 1982. Rand Corp. Pub. R–2901–HCFA.

22. See reference 12 above.

23. See reference 18 above.

24. See reference 20 above.

25. Becker, E.R., and F.A. Sloan. Utilization of hospital services: The roles of teaching, case-mix, and reimbursement. *Inquiry.* 1983; 20:248–57.

26. Markel, G.A. Hospital utilization effects of case reimbursement for medical care. In Gabel, J.R., J. Taylor, N.T. Greenspan, and M.O. Blaxall, eds.

Physicians and Financial Incentives. Washington, D.C.: U.S. Government Printing Office, 1980; 95–99.

27. See reference 1 above.

28. Epstein, A.M., S.J. Krock, and B.J. McNeil. Office laboratory tests: Perceptions of profitability. *Med. Care.* 1984; 22:160–66.

29. Epstein, A.M., C.B. Begg, and B.J. McNeil. The effects of group size on test ordering for hypertensive patients. *N. Engl. J. Med.* 1983; 309:464–68.

30. Schroeder, S.A., and J.A. Showstack. Financial incentives to perform medical procedures and laboratory tests: Illustrative models of office practice. *Med. Care.* 1978; 16:289–98.

31. Childs, A.W., and E.D. Hunter. Non-medical factors influencing use of diagnostic x-ray by physicians. *Med. Care.* 1972; 10:323–35.

32. See reference 18 above.

33. Bailey, R.M. *Clinical Laboratories and the Practice of Medicine.* Berkeley, Calif.: McCutchan Publishing Corp., 1979.

34. See reference 18 above.

35. Schicke, R.K. Economic aspects of diagnostic services in health care. *Methods Inf. Med.* 1983; 22:1–33.

36. See reference 18 above.

37. See reference 1 above.

38. Wennberg, J., and A. Gittelsohn. Variations in medical care among small areas. *Sci. Am.* 1982; 246(4):120–34.

39. Roos, N.P. Hysterectomy: Variation in rates across small areas and across physicians' practices. *Am. J. Public Health.* 1984; 74:327–35.

40. Roos, L.L., Jr. Supply, workload and utilization: A population-based analysis of surgery in rural Manitoba. *Am. J. Public Health.* 1983; 73:414–21.

41. Hardwick, D.F., P. Vertinsky, R.T. Barth, V.F. Mitchell, M. Bernstein, and I. Vertinsky. Clinical styles and motivation: A study of laboratory test use. *Med. Care.* 1975; 13:397–408.

42. Williams, S.V., J.M. Eisenberg, L.A. Pascale, and D.S. Kitz. Physicians' perceptions about unnecessary diagnostic testing. *Inquiry.* 1982; 19:363–70.

43. Campbell, D.M. Why do physicians in neonatal care units differ in their admission thresholds? *Soc. Sci. Med.* 1984; 18:365–74.

44. Pauly, M.V. Medical staff characteristics and hospital costs. *J. Hum. Resour.* 1978; 13(suppl):77–111.

45. See reference 39 above.

46. Kaluzny, A.D., J.E. Veney, and J.T. Gentry. Innovation of health services: A comparative study of hospitals and health departments. *Milbank Mem. Fund Q.* 1974; 52:51–82.

47. Kaluzny, A.D. Innovation in health system: A selective review of system characteristics and empirical research. In Abernathy, W.J., A. Sheldon, and C.K. Prahalad. *The Management of Health Care.* Cambridge, Mass.: Ballinger Publishing Co., 1974; 67–68.

48. Becker, M.H. Sociometric location and innovativeness: Reformulation and extension of the diffusion model. *Am. Sociol. Rev.* 1970; 35:267–82.

49. Rothert, M.L., D.R. Rovner, A.S. Elstein, G.B. Holzman, M.M. Holmes, and M.M. Ravitch. Differences in medical referral decisions for obesity among family practitioners, general internists, and gynecologists. *Med. Care.* 1984; 22:42–55.

50. Eisenberg, J.M. Sociological influences on decision making by clinicians. *Ann. Intern. Med.* 1979; 90:957–64.

51. See reference 1 above.

52. Gold, M. Effects of hospital-based primary care setting on internists' treatment of primary care episodes. *Health Serv. Res.* 1981; 16:383–405.

53. Gold, M., and M. Greenlick. Effect of hospital-based primary care setting on internists' use of inpatient hospital resources. *Med. Care.* 1981; 19:160–71.

54. Rosenblatt, R.A., and I.S. Moscovice. The physician as gatekeeper: Determinants of physicians' hospitalization rates. *Med. Care.* 1984; 22:150–59.

55. See reference 43 above.

56. Chu, R.C., S.V. Williams, and J.M. Eisenberg. The characteristics of stat laboratory tests. *Arch. Pathol. Lab. Med.* 1982; 106:662–65.

57. Boardman, A.E., B. Dowd, J.M. Eisenberg, et al. A model of physicians' practice attributes determination. *J. Health Econ.* 1984; 2:259–68.

58. See reference 31 above.

59. Noren, J., T. Frazier, I. Altman, and J. DeLozier. Ambulatory medical care: A comparison of internists and family-general practitioners. *N. Engl. J. Med.* 1980; 302:11–16.

60. Ernst, R. Ancillary production and the size of physicians' practice. *Inquiry.* 1976; 13:371–81.

61. Fishbane, M., and B. Starfield. Child health care in the United States: A comparison of pediatricians and general practitioners. *N. Engl. J. Med.* 1981; 305:552–56.

62. Manu, P., and S.E. Schwartz. Patterns of diagnostic testing in the academic setting: The influence of medical attendings' subspecialty training. *Soc. Sci. Med.* 1983; 17:1339–42.

63. Everett, G.D., P.F. Chang, C.S. de Blois, and T.D. Holets. A comparative study of laboratory utilization behavior on "on-service" and "off-service" house staff physicians. *Med. Care.* 1983; 21:1187–91.

64. Eisenberg, J.M., D.S. Kitz, and R.A. Webber. Development of attitudes about sharing decision making: A comparison of medical and surgical residents. *J. Health Soc. Behav.* 1983; 24:85–90.

65. Rich, E.C., T.W. Crowson, and D.P. Connelly. Evidence for an informal clinical policy resulting in high use of a very-low-yield test. *Am. J. Med.* 1985; 79:577–82.

66. Greenwald, H.P., M.L. Peterson, L.P. Garrison, et al. Interspecialty variation in office-based care. *Med. Care.* 1984; 22:14–29.

67. Eisenberg, J.M., and D. Nicklin. Use of diagnostic services by physicians in community practice. *Med. Care.* 1981; 19:297–309.

68. See reference 67 above.

69. See reference 41 above.

70. Roos, M.P., G. Flowerdew, A. Wajda, and R.B. Tate. Variations in physicians' hospitalization practices: A population-based study in Manitoba, Canada. *Am. J. Public Health.* 1986; 76:45–51.

71. Linn, L.S., J. Yager, B.D. Leake, et al. Differences in the numbers and costs of tests ordered by internists, family physicians and psychiatrists. *Inquiry.* 1984; 21:266–75.

72. See reference 49 above.

73. Dietrich, A.J., and H. Goldberg. Preventive content of adult primary care: Do generalists and subspecialists differ? *Am. J. Public Health.* 1984; 74:223–27.

74. See reference 49 above.

75. Munch, P. Economic incentives to order lab tests: Theory and evidence. In Hough, D.E., and G.I. Misek, eds. *Socioeconomic Issues of Health.* Chicago: American Medical Assoc., 1980; 59–83.

76. See reference 31 above.

77. See reference 43 above.

78. See reference 67 above.

79. Pineault, R. The effect of medical training factors on physician utilization behavior. *Med. Care.* 1977; 15:51–67.

80. Freeborn, D.K., D. Baer, M.R. Greenlick, and J.W. Bailey. Determinants of medical care utilization: Physicians' use of laboratory services. *Am. J. Public Health.* 1972; 62:846–53.

81. See reference 75 above.

82. Schroeder, S.A., K. Kenders, J.K. Cooper, and T.E. Piemme. Use of laboratory tests and pharmaceuticals: Variation among physicians and effect of cost audit on subsequent use. *J.A.M.A.* 1973; 225:969–73.

83. See reference 67 above.

84. Epstein, A.M., C.B. Begg, and B.J. McNeil. The effects of physician training and personality on test ordering for ambulatory patients. *Am. J. Public Health.* 1984; 74:1271–73.

85. See reference 43 above.

86. Goldfarb, M.G., M.C. Hornbrook, and C.S. Higgins. Determinants of hospital use: A cross-diagnostic analysis. *Med. Care.* 1983; 21:48–66.

87. See reference 48 above.

88. Estes, E.H., Jr. The behavior of health professionals: Impact on cost and quality of care. *Duke Univ. Med. Cent. Perspect.* 1983; 3:7–13.

89. Cummings, K.M., K.B. Frisof, M.J. Long, and G. Krynkiewich. The effect of price information on physicians' test ordering behavior: Ordering of diagnostic tests. *Med. Care.* 1982; 20:293.

90. Boice, J.L., and M. McGregor. Effect of residents' use of laboratory tests on hospital costs. *J. Med. Educ.* 1983; 58:61–64.

91. Applegate, W.B., M.D. Bennett, L. Chilton, B.J. Skipper, and R.E. White. Impact of a cost containment educational program on house staff ambulatory clinic charges. *Med. Care.* 1983; 21:486–96.

92. Greenland, P., A.I. Mushlin, and P.F. Griner. Discrepancies between knowledge and use of diagnostic studies in asymptomatic patients. *J. Med. Educ.* 1979; 54:863–69.

93. Cebul, R.D. Personal communication.

94. Hadsall, R.S., R.A. Freeman, and G.J. Norwood. Factors related to the prescribing of selected psychotropic drugs by primary care physicians. *Soc. Sci. Med.* 1982; 16:1747–56.

95. See reference 79 above.

96. See reference 84 above.

97. See reference 67 above.

98. See reference 75 above.

99. See reference 67 above.

100. See reference 31 above.

101. See reference 66 above.

102. See reference 68 above.

103. See reference 79 above.

104. See reference 80 above.

105. Eisenberg, J.M., and S.V. Williams. Cost containment and changing physicians' practice behavior: Can the fox learn to guard the chicken coop? *J.A.M.A.* 1981; 246:2195–2201.

106. Rothberg, D.L. Regional variations in hospital use: Introduction and overview. In Rothberg, D.L., ed. *Regional Variations in Hospital Use.* Lexington, Mass.: Lexington Books, 1982; 1–20.

107. See reference 1 above.

108. Fuchs, V.R., and J.P. Newhouse. National Bureau of Economic Research Conference on the economics of physician and patient behavior: The conference and unresolved problems. *J. Hum. Resour.* 1978; 13(suppl):1–18.

109. Freidson, E. *Profession of Medicine: A Study of the Sociology of Applied Knowledge.* New York: Dodd, Mead & Co., 1970.

110. See reference 50 above.

111. See reference 94 above.

112. Long, M.J., K.M. Cummings, and K.B. Frisof. The role of perceived price in physicians' demand for diagnostic tests. *Med. Care.* 1983; 21:243–50.

113. See reference 40 above.

114. Jones, K.R. The influence of the attending physician on indirect graduate medical education costs. *J. Med. Educ.* 1984; 59:789–98.

115. Garber, A.M., V.R. Fuchs, and J.F. Silverman. Case mix, cost and outcomes. *N. Engl. J. Med.* 1984; 310:1231–37.

116. See reference 115 above.

117. See reference 54 above.

118. Luft, H.S. Variations in clinical practice patterns. *Arch. Intern. Med.* 1983; 143:1861–62.

119. Luft, H.S. How do health-maintenance organizations achieve their "savings"? *N. Engl. J. Med.* 1978; 298:1336–43.

120. LoGerfo, J.P. Organizational and financial influences on patterns of surgical care. *Surg. Clin. North Am.* 1982; 62:677–84.

121. Hlatky, M.A., K.L. Lee, E.H. Botvinick, and B.H. Brundage. Diagnostic test use in different practice settings: A controlled comparison. *Arch. Intern. Med.* 1983; 143:1886–89.

122. Yelin, E.H., C.J. Henke, J.S. Kramer, et al. A comparison of the treatment of rheumatoid arthritis in health maintenance organizations and fee-for-service practices. *N. Engl. J. Med.* 1985; 312:962–67.

123. Manning, W.G. *The Use of Pathology Services: A Comparison of Fee-for-Service and a Prepaid Group Practice.* Santa Monica, Calif.: Rand Corp., January 1983. Rand Corp. Pub. R–2919–HCFA.

124. Pineault, R. The effect of prepaid group practice on physicians' utilization behavior. *Med. Care.* 1976; 14:121–36.

125. Dorsey, J.L. Use of diagnostic resources in health maintenance organizations and fee-for-service practice settings. *Arch. Intern. Med.* 1983; 143:1863–65.

126. Hartzema, A.G., and D.B. Christensen. Nonmedical factors associated with the prescribing volume among family practitioners in an HMO. *Med. Care.* 1983; 21:990–1000.

127. Zelnio, R.N. The interaction among the criteria physicians use when prescribing. *Med. Care.* 1982; 20:277–85.

128. See reference 124 above.

129. See reference 29 above.

130. See reference 125 above.

131. Eddy, D.M. Clinical policies and the quality of clinical practice. *N. Engl. J. Med.* 1982; 307:343–47.

132. Tatchell, M. Measuring hospital output: A review of the service mix and case mix approaches. *Soc. Sci. Med.* 1983; 17:871–83.

133. See reference 86 above.

134. Hornbrook, M.C., and M.G. Goldfarb. A partial test of a hospital behavioral model. *Soc. Sci. Med.* 1983; 17:667–80.

135. DesHarnais, S., N.M. Kibe, and S. Barbus. Blue Cross and Blue Shield of Michigan Hospital Laboratory On-Site Review Project. *Inquiry.* 1983; 20:328–33.

136. Read, J.L., R.S. Stern, L.A. Thibodeau, D.E. Geer, Jr., and H. Klapholz.

Variation in antenatal testing over time and between clinic settings. *J.A.M.A.* 1983; 249:1605–9.

137. Stross, J.K., and G.G. Bole. Evaluation of a continuing education program in rheumatoid arthritis. *Arthritis Rheum.* 1980; 23:846–49.

138. Stross, J.K., R.G. Hiss, C.M. Watts, W.K. Davis, and R. McDonald. Continuing education in pulmonary disease for primary-care physicians. *Am. Rev. Respir. Dis.* 1983; 127:739–46.

139. See reference 38 above.

140. Flood, A.B., W.R. Scott, W. Ewy, and W.H. Forrest, Jr. Effectiveness in professional organizations: The impact of surgeons and surgical staff organizations on the quality of care in hospitals. *Health Serv. Res.* 1982; 17:341–66.

141. Rhee, S.O., R.D. Luke, and M.B. Culverwell. Influence of client/colleague dependence on physician performance in patient care. *Med. Care.* 1980; 18:829–41.

142. See reference 80 above.

143. See reference 137 above.

144. See reference 138 above.

145. Coleman, J.S., E. Katz, and H. Menzel. *Medical Innovation: A Diffusion Study.* New York: Bobbs-Merrill, 1966.

146. Coleman, J., H. Menzel, and E. Katz. Social process in physicians' adoption of a new drug. *J. Chronic Dis.* 1959; 9:1–9.

147. Greer, A.L. Advances in the study of diffusion of innovation in health care organizations. *Milbank Mem. Fund Q.* 1977; 55:505–62.

148. Greer, A.L. Medical technology and professional dominance theory. *Soc. Sci. Med.* 1984; 10:809–17.

149. Anderson, J.G., and S.J. Jay. Utilization of computers in clinical practice—the role of physician networks: Preliminary communication. *J. R. Soc. Med.* 1983; 76:45–52.

150. See reference 145 above.

151. Winkler, J.D., K.N. Lohr, and R.H. Brook. Persuasive communication and medical technology assessment. *Arch. Intern. Med.* 1985; 145:314–17.

152. Rogers, F.M. *Diffusion of Innovations.* New York: Free Press, 1983.

153. Avorn, J., M. Chen, and R. Hartley. Scientific versus commercial sources of influence on the prescribing behavior of physicians. *Am. J. Med.* 1982; 73:4–8.

3

The Physician as the Patient's Agent

Levels of utilization of medical services undoubtedly depend in large part on the self-fulfilling motivations, desires, and styles of the individual physician. Practice patterns are profoundly influenced by physicians' desires for income, their personal characteristics, their desired practice styles, and the influence of peers and practice settings, as was discussed in the previous chapter. However, the literature on practice patterns also demonstrates that physicians serve as their patients' agents and that their practice patterns are driven in large part by a desire to act in their patients' best interests. Physician decision making is a complex interaction of attempts to satisfy the physicians' personal desires and those of the patient. In fact, the literature suggests an intertwining of these two sets of desires, each of which can be described as a multiattribute utility function (an effort to satisfy simultaneously a number of goals, some of which are conflicting). A substantial part of the physician's satisfaction with practice is fulfilled by serving successfully as the patient's advocate.

Although as much as 90 percent of medical care utilization is initiated by physicians, almost all of this care seems to represent services that patients would have chosen if the patients had sufficient knowledge to make the decision alone [1, 2]. By our definition of physician inducement (inducement, as opposed to initiation, is prescription of services that a well-informed consumer would not want to use), physicians appear to maintain remarkable fidelity to their roles as their patients' agents. It could be that differences in physicians' practice styles simply reflect differences in their clienteles. Alternatively, it may be that patients choose physicians whose practice styles are consistent with their own desires, and that the wide variations among physicians simply serve to satisfy the heterogenous preferences of the population. Whichever is the cause and whichever is the effect, physicians' practice styles and the desires of their patients are clearly related.

Patients who do not agree with their physicians' prescriptions certainly have the option of refusing to comply with them—missing follow-up appointments, refusing surgery, or not taking prescribed medications. A portion of noncompliance by patients may be due to this difference between what well-informed patients would choose to use and what physicians have chosen to prescribe. However, a substantial portion of patients' failure to comply is certainly due to their incomplete knowledge or to psychological factors, such as difficulty understanding the importance of the doctor's prescription to their own well-being.

The physician's role as the patient's agent has six components. First, the physician will seek to defend the patient's economic well-being. However, because the physician's own economic well-being often requires that the patient pay for medical care out of pocket, the physician's self-interest may be in conflict with this desire to serve the patient's interest. Second, clinical factors certainly play a role in medical decision making, and the physician's role as healer is central to the doctor-patient relationship. Preventing, diagnosing, and treating disease are the physician's principal charges, and to serve as the patient's agent, the physician must ensure that his medical decisions represent good clinical practice. Third, doctors will be influenced by their patients' preferences, which are manifest through patient demand for medical care. The patient's preferences and expectations are also the driving forces behind a fourth influence on medical decision making: the concern about possible malpractice suits and the resultant practice of defensive medicine. Fifth, the patient's characteristics and, sixth, the patient's convenience affect the services that the physician prescribes.

The Patient's Economic Agent

Although there is substantial evidence that physicians have poor knowledge of the price of medical care services (not to mention their misunderstanding of its true cost), the price that a patient must pay for services does seem to affect physicians' patterns of prescribing services [4–7]. In addition to being poorly informed about the price of services, physicians may not appreciate the individual preferences of their patients [8]. Research in medical decision making suggests that physicians, using their understanding of what their patients want (which may mean the doctor's best guess), sometimes arrive at different plans for diagnosis or treatment than the patients would actually prefer. The literature from decision sciences offers several formal techniques with which doctors can improve their ability to incorporate patients' values into the decision-making process, but few physicians are likely to use these methods in day-to-day patient care [9–11].

Despite their lack of knowledge of price and patient preference, physicians do respond to differences in the price of medical care by varying their utilization of services. In chapter 1, evidence was provided to show how doctors may adjust their utilization to maintain income, resulting in decreased use rates with higher fees and vice versa. In addition to this self-interested response to changes in fees, physicians may also consider the portion of the fee that is paid by the patient out of pocket. In fact, the price elasticity of demand for medical care (that is, lower demand at higher prices) may operate through the physician serving as the patient's agent [12]. This paradigm places the physician on the demand side of the equation rather than the supply side and exemplifies the dual role that physicians play.

Some evidence suggests that the change in the number of ambulatory visits to physicians (which correlates with changes in the out-of-pocket price to patients for the visits) is due, at least in part, to changes in the number of physician-initiated visits. In one study, a 10 percent increase in out-of-pocket price was correlated with a decrease of 0.15 visits per patient per year (about 5 percent of the average of 3.5 visits per year). Interestingly, patient-initiated visits did not change, suggesting that patients themselves are not sensitive to differences in the out-of-pocket price they face when initiating demand for physician care. The decrease in visits was due to a smaller number of physician-initiated visits (which are mostly follow-up visits and may be more discretionary). However, other studies have also shown a response of patient-initiated visits to the out-of-pocket price of care [13].

Physicians also seem to be influenced by cost in the number of tests they prescribe. Hoey and colleagues [14] showed that 24 percent to 38 percent of test ordering is sensitive to the price of the diagnostic test, depending on the physician's level of experience. The remainder of test-ordering decisions seems to be driven by clinical considerations. The proportion of responses to test-ordering choices that are sensitive to price seems to be inversely related to the physician's clinical experience, with medical students being the most influenced, interns and residents being intermediate, and staff physicians being the least. In part, this inverse relation may have been due to decisions by staff physicians to order fewer tests regardless of price, leaving fewer tests to be ordered and influenced by price. Perhaps staff physicians, being more clinically experienced, did not feel that the tests would be useful, no matter how low the cost.

Contradictory evidence comes from the Rand studies of factors affecting laboratory test use [15]. In both a survey of physicians and the large Rand Health Insurance Experiment, no clear relationship was evident between the patient's out-of-pocket cost and the probability that the physician would perform a test during an office visit. On the other hand, a trend was seen in the survey toward physicians ordering fewer tests for uninsured patients. The Rand researchers explain these contradictory results as potentially being due to the confounding influence of patients' clinical status. Because patients with generous insurance benefits are more likely to consult a physician and therefore may, on average, be less sick than patients on other health plans who seek care, their likelihood of needing to have tests done during a visit might be lower. Again, the difficulty of controlling for case mix and severity of disease obscures our ability to understand how other factors influence physicians' practice patterns.

In another study, when physicians underestimated the price of a test, they tended to order more of them and when they overestimated the price, they ordered fewer: the greater the propensity to underestimate, the greater the number of tests ordered; the greater the propensity to overestimate, the fewer the number of tests ordered [16]. Although these were perceived prices rather than actual prices that influenced decision making, the results of this study do suggest that physicians act as their patients' economic agents in the prescription of diagnostic tests. Similar results have been found in studies of drug prescribing and dental procedures [17, 18]. The prescription of hospital services for self-paying patients is substantially less than that for Medicaid patients [19]. This finding may reflect an effort by the physician to practice more cost-effective medicine for the self-paying patient.

In addition to the patient's out-of-pocket cost for medical services, physicians take into account the opportunity costs of medical care to their patients. Physicians, when prescribing services, consider the amount of time that patients will spend to receive medical care and therefore, time that patients will miss from productive activities such as work [20, 21].

This behavior of the physician as the patient's economic agent may not be entirely altruistic. The physician may serve as the patient's advocate in order to retain the patient as a client. By this argument, the more competitive the medical market is, the more the physician should act as the patient's agent. In addition to reducing out-of-pocket expenses for the patient, the physician who acts as the patient's economic agent by reducing the number of nonphysician expenses, such as tests, drugs, or hospital days, may also be making it possible for the patient to spend more of his health care dollar on physician fees [22].

Even if patients do not actually spend more money on doctors' fees when they save on hospitalization and ancillary services, it may be in the physicians' economic interest to practice in a cost-effective manner, even in fee-for-service practice. Patients who are dissatisfied with the cost of their care may decide to find a less costly physician, assuming that they have access to the data that would allow them to make this decision (which is rarely the case except by word of mouth). However, with increased attention to health care costs by third-party payers and employers, and with brokered and managed care being more common, the pressure on doctors to save money for their patients is becoming less subtle. Employers and payers are increasingly interested in obtaining data about the costs incurred by different physicians; they are also making these data available to the doctors' patients and giving patients incentives to spend less on their health care.

The Patient's Clinical Agent

In addition to serving as the patients' agents with regard to the cost of medical care, physicians serve as the patients' agents in ensuring the quality of care and the provision of services necessary for the patients' health. Whether this behavior is intended to retain satisfied patients or occurs because it is consistent with physicians' professional ethos (and because they have personal utility for their satisfaction with the quality of their work), the point remains that a large portion of medical care utilization occurs as a result of physicians acting as the patient's agent in clinical matters. The unifying hypothesis is that physicians do have personal utility for their patients' benefit.

Physicians' concern for their patients' health has been shown to be a major determinant of their utilization patterns. Clinical factors are the strongest predictor of physician-initiated office visits [23, 24], and patients' health status is an important predictor of the use of hospital beds [25]. In the decision to recommend surgery to patients, the physician's belief that surgery will help is a major factor [26, 27]. Certainly, the physician's personal beliefs and enthusiasm (whether correct or not) are important influences in the prescription of other medical services as well, such as psychotropic drugs [28]. In fact, the most important variable in physicians' choice of drugs is the perception of their effectiveness and risk [29]. Although price does influence physicians' use of diagnostic tests, clinical considerations are substantially more important and the importance of clinical factors increases with the greater clinical maturity of the decision maker [30].

Clinicians writing about the differences in physician utilization and the influences on their practice patterns assume that any doctor would want to give better care if it were possible [31]. Economists, while they naturally tend to emphasize economic factors in determining practice patterns, recognize the utility to the clinician of providing quality care, independent of its financial consequences [32, 33]. Pauly's compromise position describes the merger of the philosophies of physician-as-perfect-agent and physician-as-income-seeker [34]. He describes physicians as "partially benevolent oligopolists." Assuming all other things being equal, he suggests, physicians would rather tell the truth to their patients and serve as perfect agents. However, they would be willing to surrender some accuracy for some income.

Because physicians' beliefs about the effectiveness and risk of medical services are of such central importance, the certainty with which they hold these beliefs is critical in determining their levels of utilization. Many investigators have described the importance of clinical uncertainty in physicians' practice patterns. Eddy has emphasized the ambiguity inherent in defining the difference between normal and abnormal, characterizing disease entities, collecting accurate data, evaluating diagnostic tests, and measuring outcomes [35]. This uncertainty may exist because the knowledge simply is not available. In many areas of medical practice, even physicians who are experts in the field and who have complete mastery of the available information about the usefulness and risk of a service would agree that the data are insufficient about many problems to allow them to arrive at firm conclusions. Alternatively, the uncertainty may exist because the physicians do not have access to the available evidence or are unable to make use of the available information appropriately. Even if the data were sufficient and the physicians were aware of the data and able to process the information effectively, they might not understand their patient's preferences.

Because physicians as perfect agents would make the same decision as their patients would make if the patients were as knowledgeable as they, physicians as perfect agents must know their patients' values, willingness to accept risk, and decision-making process. The task is awesome and offers a challenge to physicians who want to act on behalf of their patients.

Because uncertainty seems inevitable, it must be considered as an element in medical decision making [36]. The clinical ambiguity of a case has important effects on the amount of testing that physicians perform [37], and incomplete or outdated medical knowledge helps to explain variations in drug-prescribing practices [38–40]. Much of the work by Wennberg and colleagues in studying small-area variations in surgery leads to the conclusion that uncertainty is a key factor in these variations [41–45]. Wider variation in surgical rates has been found for children when the indications for surgery were poorly defined by the available clinical evidence [46]. The same relationship between clinical beliefs, or certainty, and utilization exists for prevention. A physician's belief in the value of preventive measures is a major determinant in utilization [47]. These results suggest that variation in practice patterns is expected, not only for statistical and behavioral reasons, but also for reasons of clinical uncertainty.

John Wennberg, the major proponent of uncertainty as a cause of variation in medical practice, has identified three sources of uncertainty [48]. First, uncertainty stems in part from difficulties in classifying a particular patient, so that the probabilities of disease, extent of disease, prognosis, and treatment outcomes cannot be reasonably ascertained. Second, information commonly does not exist on the probabilities of treatment outcomes under controlled circumstances. Finally, uncertainty exists even when patients are appropriately classified and outcome probabilities are known, because the values of the physician, who makes vicarious decisions, may not correspond to the patient's values.

Still a fourth form of uncertainty exists for physicians who properly classify their patients, ascribe accurate probabilities of outcomes, and understand their patients' values. Even if these first three sources of ignorance are reduced or eliminated, medical care remains a risky process. The fact that outcomes can be expressed as probabilities means that we remain uncertain about how an individual patient will turn out. In other words, uncertainty in medical practice includes more than ignorance; even if group statistics are available, the outcome will continue to be uncertain for each patient as long as medical care is a stochastic, or probabilistic, process.

Wennberg's formulation of uncertainty as a major factor in the variation among practitioners is consistent with the work of British sociologist Michael Bloor. Observing that otolaryngologists varied widely in their decisions about tonsillectomy, Bloor has concluded that specialists differ in several ways: their willingness to tolerate various levels of certitude, their indications for surgery, and even their conceptualizations of what a particular disease is [49–51]. Since certain disease entities may be less well defined than others, physicians' definitions of the disease may be relatively abstract. Bloor recollects the relevant work of an eighteenth-century philosopher, Bishop George Berkeley, who argued that the conceptions that men frame are not usually expressed as abstractions but rather as particularized and specific generalities [52]. Therefore, Bloor suggests, the ideas that physicians hold and the way they deal with the abstractions and uncertainties of medical care will influence their practice patterns. He concludes that physicians establish routines as a way of dealing with uncertainties, and that they are influenced by the routines of their colleagues. Their main source of information about the routines of colleagues will be indirect, through casual and nonspecific conversations.

An example of the way that these informal routines are communicated is found in the study of housestaff use of cerebrospinal fluid cultures for tuberculosis, in which medical and neurologic residents were found to differ substantially from pediatric residents [53]. Rich and colleagues describe the establishment of clinical policies, such as the use of tuberculosis cultures, as "categorical," as distinguished from "probabilistic," reasoning. Categorical decision making gives an unambiguous result even when the optimal choice is not clear. Whether right or wrong, categorical reasoning is much easier for physicians to deal with than probabilistic decision making, which requires identification of alternative courses of action, possible outcomes, the probabilities of each, and the utility of each outcome. It is no small wonder that local clinical rules of thumb often guide practice in areas of high uncertainty, and that as a result there are wide interregional differences in practice patterns for these clinical problems, especially given the discomfort with which most physicians deal with probabilities and uncertainty.

Another way in which uncertainty enters the medical decision-making process is through the patient. Patient demand plays an important role in medical care utilization, so the patient's own uncertainty is likely to be important. If patients are uncertain about the meaning of disease classifications, the probabilities of various clinical outcomes, or the value (that is, utility) of the possible outcomes, they will demand varying amounts of care. For the same reasons that Wennberg suggests variation can be limited by reducing physician uncertainty [54], the same principle should hold for patients.

As physicians consider the possible outcomes of medical care and the probabilities, they may well choose to err on the side of conservatism if they are averse to risk (or perceive their patients to be). Whether physicians are high or low users of services in these uncertain situations (which may be the rule and not the exception in medical care) may depend on whether they are more averse to risk from the unknown natural history of disease or from the unknown adverse side effects of diagnosis and treatment. This aversion to risk may be one reason that, as physicians become more comfortable with a new diagnostic technology and more certain of its value, patients with lower risk of disease get tested [55].

In emphasizing the importance of uncertainty in medical decision making, Wennberg proposes that differences in the rates of use for the same service are more accurately characterized as the effect on consumption by different beliefs that are held by individual physicians, rather than as demand originating in patients or as self-serving behavior of physicians acting in narrow economic self-interest [56]. In responding to the paper [57] from which this book evolved, Wennberg suggests that uncertainty is the most important factor influencing physician behavior, even in the category of the physician as self-interested practitioner.

Given this uncertainty, it is not surprising that physicians seeking to provide optimal care are influenced by forces outside the doctor-patient interaction. In addition to the influences of peers and professional leadership, commercial sources also offer substantial influences. Whereas these influences may be less important than scientific influences such as published research and review articles [58], the role of drug company representatives ("detail men") as purveyors of scientific information, albeit potentially biased information, is substantial [59–61]. Data indicate that more knowledgeable physicians, as measured by board certification, are less dependent on commercial messages than are physicians who are not board certified [62].

Despite the importance of uncertainty in medical decision making, we would be mistaken to explain away the variation in medical practice simply (or even principally) as a function of uncertainty. This approach is too narrow; it underestimates the complexity of medical decision making and the multiple influences on it. Because all physicians face uncertainty in their practices (but admittedly to different degrees), the ways that they respond to the uncertainty offer clues to the other factors that influence their practices. Uncertain clinical situations may well be the ones in which the economic, sociologic, and psychologic factors most influence the decisions that are made. But even if uncertainty were substantially reduced, these other factors would (and should) play an important role in medical decision making.

Even with perfect information, physicians would not all make identical decisions. Elstein and colleagues have described the cognitive factors that influence physician decision making as they have been revealed by research in the fields of information processing, social judgement, and decision theory [63]. For example, decision theory suggests that physicians would be expected to make different decisions for their patients if the prevalence of certain diseases were different in their practices. The predictive value of a diagnostic test depends on the prevalence of disease in the population as well as the test's sensitivity and specificity. Even when patients seem to have the same clinical characteristics, the degree to which a positive or negative test result predicts the presence or absence of disease depends on the prevalence of disease in the doctor's practice. This relationship of predictive value and prevalence, which is established by Bayesian decision theory (a mathematical approach to revising probabilities on the basis of new information), may explain why physicians appear to differ in their thresholds for testing and treatment. If the prevalence of disease in their practices differ, they should use tests and their results differently.

Differences in the prevalence of disease in different populations may explain why Hlatky and coworkers found that with similar cardiologic cases, doctors in health maintenance organizations chose to order nuclear cardiac scanning for 47 percent of patients, whereas community practitioners did so for 67 percent and university hospital clinicians did so for 72 percent [64]. Because the prevalence of disease is different in these populations, these differences in utilization may be clinically appropriate. These physicians may have been acting in a manner consistent with serving as the patient's clinical agent.

It should not be surprising, in fact it should be expected, that the severity of disease usually seen in a practice will have an effect on utilization patterns, even when case mix is controlled. In part, this difference in use is due to the different probabilities of disease for seemingly similar patients in different practices as a result of the bias of referral and patient self-selection. A patient with chest pain who chooses to seek evaluation in the office of a cardiologist who supervises an angiography laboratory is more likely to have angina than a patient with apparently the same clinical story who visits a generalist's office.

Because of the complexity of medical decision making, the last ten years have witnessed increasing interest in methods of improving decision making. Medical decision analysis and cost-benefit/cost-effectiveness analysis have been applied to a number of clinical problems and are used increasingly by researchers to recommend optimal strategies of patient care. By providing a framework for identifying the nature of the problem (and a structured way of approaching it) along with a quantitative method for incorporating probabilities and the values of different outcomes, these systems of problem solving offer help to the doctor who is uncertain not because of ignorance but because of difficulty in putting the data together in a sensible way. These methods of decision analysis and cost-benefit/cost-effectiveness analysis also are useful in identifying the key areas of ignorance, where better data are needed about probabilities and outcomes. While these data can sometimes be obtained from the published literature or from experts, sometimes their absence inspires new research to answer the question.

Although medical decision-making methods have been prominent in the medical literature for several years, they are only beginning to influence actual clinical decision making. New programs are being developed to teach clinicians about these approaches to clinical problem solving, and their early results suggest that physicians can learn these techniques even in short courses [65]. Although these methods have been criticized as being inapplicable to real clinical stituations because of the paucity of accurate data about the necessary probabilities and outcomes, the truth is that doctors are already using these imprecise data in their present decisions [66]. The formal approaches simply offer a systematic way of using the best data available and allow the doctor to understand better whether different assumptions will alter the optimal decision.

Patient Demand

Considering the physician's role as the patient's agent and the desire to act on behalf of the patient, it is not surprising that patient demand has an important effect on the utilization of services. Although patient demand is frequently listed as a cause of overutilization [67, 68], variation in utilization due to patients' preferences may be desirable. The simplistic view of the need for medical care as a biological phenomenon neglects differences in patients' tastes and desires, the prices they pay, and the resources available to them [69]. Because none of these factors is absolute and because judgements about them are value laden, it is dangerous to suggest that excess demand (that is, potential or real desire for medical care that is not being received) ipso facto implies the potential for unnecessary or inappropriate care.

To the extent that patient demand can be generated by altering patients' beliefs, the information that physicians provide patients gives them potential control over the amount and type of patient demand for medical services. Pauly and Satterthwaite have suggested that with increasing physician density, physicians can become more monopolistic because information sharing among consumers is difficult when there are large numbers of physicians [70]. On the other hand, it is in just these areas of high physician density that consumers have access to a multitude of other information about their health, including the mass media, community groups, and organizations involved in health education. These alternative sources of information may counter the monopolistic tendency that Pauly and Satterthwaite attribute to areas with many doctors.

Whether patient demand is caused by intrinsic preferences of patients or by the persuasion of physicians, evidence shows that it has an important role in influencing physicians' prescription of medical care. Although the factors underlying patient demand are poorly understood, the influence of patient demand on physicians' drug-prescribing patterns is well documented [71–73]. Patient demand has also been described for surgery [74] in the case of hysterectomy [75], for referrals [76], and for diagnostic tests [77, 78]. For example, for two-thirds of patients who had upper gastrointestinal radiographic series, the patient's expectation that the study would be done was a factor in its ordering [79]. Rothert and colleagues found that the patient's desire for referral to an endocrinologist for the work-up of obesity was the most important factor in the decision to refer [80].

Reviewing the factors that influence patients' utilization of medical care, Hulka and Wheat reached three conclusions about patient demand that suggest the importance of health status and the patient's perception of it [81]. First, health status is the most important determinant of utilization; health status or other variables that describe the need for medical care explain the greatest amount of variability in utilization. Second, patients' perception of need is most likely to influence first contact care, whereas physicians are more important in affecting follow-up visits, procedures performed, and hospital admission rates. Third, from the methodologic perspective, health status requires more emphasis in research to ensure that the relevant measures be selected and find their way into the multivariate models of medical care utilization.

On the other hand, the patient's desire for medical services is not entirely due to clinical factors. For example, the desire to be admitted to the hospital may be due to the absence of social support systems at home [82]. Differences in utilization among communities may reflect differences in pooled preferences of their residents, which are translated into differences in patient demand [83, 84]. These differences in demand could explain some variation in utilization of medical care among small areas.

Despite the evidence that patient demand already influences physicians' prescription of medical services, data also suggest that physicians should be more sensitive to their patients' wishes. Being more responsive to patients' perceived needs may produce higher quality care. In descriptive research, elicitation of patient requests and explicit expectations has been associated with the enhancement of various health outcomes [85].

In an effort to improve physicians' understanding of patients' desires, Uhlmann and colleagues have recently called for a more explicit definition of patient demand [86]. They emphasize the difference between patients' expectations and patients' desires. Patients' desires are wishes regarding medical care and, in contrast to expectations, they primarily reflect a valuation, a perception, that a given event is wanted. An event may be desired but not expected; for example, a patient may want, but not expect, a disease to be cured. Conversely, an outcome may be expected but not desired.

Defensive Medicine

When community physicians are asked why diagnostic services are overused, a frequent response is that they fear malpractice suits and, as a result, they practice defensively to avoid them [87]. This suggestion of defensive medicine is a special case of the physicians' response to patient demand. Because of the belief that patients will sue if they are not satisfied with the outcome of their care, physicians say that they alter their utilization patterns as well as their advice, explanations, and choice of patients. Higher premiums for malpractice insurance may have led to increased testing, although this argument would support the target income hypothesis more readily than it would support the idea of defensive medicine [88].

Despite the perception of physicians that defensive medicine is an important factor in determining their practice patterns, little data support their assertion. Garg and colleagues found fear of malpractice suits to be less of a problem than was thought to be the case, although they suggested that 8 percent to 15 percent of laboratory and radiographic testing is due to defensive medicine [89]. A major study of the use of diagnostic radiology found that the practice of defensive medicine was not a major factor [90]. Even for skull radiographic examinations of emergency room patients, defensive medicine only explained about 11 percent of utilization. Others have estimated that only 1 percent of laboratory tests are due to defensive medicine and that only 2 percent of malpractice suits are due to inadequate testing [91, 92]. An analysis of defensive medicine by the staff of the *Duke Law Journal* also showed that defensive medicine was much less extensive than was generally believed [93]. Others have also suggested that the practice of defensive medicine is not a major cause of the rapidly increasing numbers of medical services prescribed by physicians [94, 95]. Perhaps this excuse is just a convenient, oversimplified scapegoat that points responsibility away from the medical community.

In fact, the organized medical community is often the one that cries loudest about defensive medicine. For example, a task force of the American Medical Association (AMA) has claimed that defensive medicine costs $15.1 billion annually in the United States [96]. These calculations were based on AMA surveys that suggested that 27.2 percent of doctors provide some additional treatment procedures as a response to the increased risk of a professional liability action, and an assumption that the average gross income for U.S. physicians was $200,000 per year. Therefore, the AMA proposes that because about one-quarter of all physician billings are due to defensive medicine (the AMA survey actually reported that 27.2 percent of doctors reported *some* defensive practices), the cost of defensive medicine would average $50,000 per doctor annually, or $15.1 billion nationally. Unfortunately, this kind of statistical legerdemain discredits other arguments the profession may make about the effect of malpractice on the cost of medical care.

With individual physicians facing startling malpractice premiums, it is inevitable that some of these costs will be passed on to the consumer (either by higher prices or induced demand). In most of New York State, the annual premium for neurosurgeons in early 1985 was $44,401; for obstetricians, $32,261; and for orthopedic surgeons, $37,643 [97]. Doctors claim that they are leaving these practices and either retiring or entering general practice (despite not having been trained for primary care) [98]. Few would argue that this is the best or most efficient way to deal with the oversupply of surgical specialists.

As the number of suits increases, defensive medicine will likely play a more important part in medical decision making, even if the number of services added does not approach the claim of over 25 percent by the AMA. Until better data are available about the real effect of malpractice suits (and fear of them) on physician behavior, there is little likelihood of more constructive dialogue.

Patient Characteristics

A number of studies have demonstrated that different patients are treated differently, even when their medical problems are identical. A variety of patient characteristics, such as social class, age, sex, income, physical appearance, and ethnic background, have been correlated with different recommendations and behaviors by physicians [99, 100]. Unfortunately, most of these studies have not investigated the reasons underlying these differences in the prescription of services for patients with different characteristics, but the differences are likely due, in some way, to the physician's role as self-interested practitioner or as the patient's agent. Patients' personal characteristics may affect their ability to pay for care, their values, their likelihood of having disease, or their aversion to risk, and thereby influence the doctor who is trying to act as the patient's agent. Conversely, patients' personal characteristics could influence the physician's expected income or pleasure with style of practice. For these reasons, it is difficult to interpret the meaning of different practice patterns for patients of different ages [101–103], sex [104–106], socioeconomic group [107], or race [108].

For example, patients from the lower socioeconomic class are diagnosed as having aberrant behavior more often than are middle-class patients, but they are less often referred for psychiatric treatment. When treated, they are seen for a briefer duration and with less intensity, even when the presumed disease is the same. In one emergency room study, blacks were more often admitted to a ward service while white patients were assigned to private practitioners. These assignments were made by clerks, who were black, rather than by physicians. Patients' physical appearances also affect medical decision making, and health professionals are more likely to perform heroic measures on patients whom they perceive as contributing more to society [109].

Although personal characteristics of patients are important when studying differences among physicians in utilization patterns, patient characteristics are probably important only as indicators of more fundamental motivators of physician behavior. Because patient characteristics are so closely correlated with other factors, studies of physician behavior that completely control for patient characteristics run the risk of what epidemiologists describe as "overcontrol" unless the variables of interest still vary among the remaining patients. For example, physicians' responses to patients' ability to pay for medical care may be important but could be obscured if all patients in a study were of the same socioeconomic status and had the same insurance coverage.

Convenience

The convenience of the patient (and the physician) may also influence utilization patterns. British physicians refer patients for laboratory testing more often if the patients are close to the testing site than if they are far [110]. Convenience may also have contributed to the observation that diagnostic testing depends in part on the availability of facilities for certain tests [111]. However, like the inverse relationship between the time a patient will need to travel to the doctor's office for a follow-up visit and the frequency of follow-up visits that are prescribed, economic factors probably interact with the desire for convenience. Patients who must travel farther for diagnostic testing are likely to incur larger travel costs and are likely to have greater opportunity costs in doing so (for example, time lost from work).

Whether for the patient's convenience or the physician's economic benefit, a number of manufacturers have produced laboratory testing equipment for doctors' offices. These tests can be done on site and results can be made available quickly, so the in-office laboratory does have some advantages for the patients' convenience. Obviously this convenience could be offset by poorer quality tests if care is not taken by those in the doctor's office who are performing the tests.

As the list of factors that influence doctors' decisions grows longer, it becomes clearer that the process is a complex one. No single factor, be it economic benefit of the doctor or uncertainty in medical decision making, suffices to explain the variation in medical practice. Nor are the doctor and patient the only parties to the process. Their interaction occurs in the context of a social milieu that at the same time influences the decisions that are made and demands that the greater good of society as a whole be considered when resources are used for the individual patient.

References

1. Wilensky, G.R., and L.F. Rossiter. The relative importance of physician-induced demand for medical care. *Milbank Mem. Fund Q.* 1983; 61:252–77.

2. Rossiter, L.F., and G.R. Wilensky. A reexamination of the use of physician services: The role of physician-initiated demand. *Inquiry.* 1983; 20:162–72.

3. Cummings, K.M., K.B. Frisof, M.J. Long, and G. Krynkiewich. The effect of price information on physicians' test ordering behavior: Ordering of diagnostic tests. *Med. Care.* 1982; 20:293.

4. Eisenberg, J.M., and S.V. Williams. Cost containment and changing physicians' practice behavior: Can the fox learn to guard the chicken coop? *J.A.M.A.* 1981; 246:2195–2201.

5. Long, M.J., K.M. Cummings, and K.B. Frisof. The role of perceived price in physicians' demand for diagnostic tests. *Med. Care.* 1983; 21:243–50.

6. Hoey, J., J.M. Eisenberg, W.O. Spitzer, and D. Thomas. Physician sensitivity to the price of diagnostic tests: A U.S.–Canadian analysis. *Med. Care.* 1982; 20:302–7.

7. Cohen, D.I., P. Jones, B. Littenberg, and D. Neuhauser. Does cost information availability reduce physician test usage? A randomized clinical trial with unexpected findings. *Med. Care.* 1982; 20:286–92.

8. Pauly, M.V. *Doctors and Their Workshops.* Chicago: National Bureau of Economic Research, The University of Chicago Press, 1980.

9. Christensen-Szalanski, J.J.J. Discount functions and the measurement of patient values: Women's decisions during childbirth. *Med. Decis. Making.* 1984; 4:47–48.

10. McNeil, B.J., R. Weichselbaum, and S.G. Pauker. Fallacy of the five year survival in lung cancer. *N. Engl. J. Med.* 1978; 299:1397–1401.

11. McNeil, B.J., B. Weichselbaum, and S.G. Pauker. Speech and survival: Tradeoffs between quality and quantity of life in laryngeal cancer. *N. Engl. J. Med.* 1981; 305:982–87.

12. See reference 8 above.

13. See reference 2 above.

14. See reference 6 above.

15. Danzon, P.M., W.G. Manning, and M.S. Marquis. Factors affecting laboratory use and prices. *Health Care Financing Rev.* 1984; 5:23–32.

16. See reference 5 above.

17. Bailit, H.L., and J. Clive. The development of dental practice profiles. *Med. Care.* 1981; 19:30–46.

18. Zelnio, R.N. The interaction among the criteria physicians use when prescribing. *Med. Care.* 1982; 20:277–85.

19. Becker, E.R., and F.A. Sloan. Utilization of hospital services: The roles of teaching, case mix, and reimbursement. *Inquiry.* 1983; 20:248–57.

20. See reference 2 above.

21. Goldfarb, M.G., M.C. Hornbrook, and C.S. Higgins. Determinants of hospital use: A cross-diagnostic analysis. *Med. Care.* 1983; 21:48–66.

22. See reference 8 above.

23. See reference 1 above.

24. See reference 2 above.

25. See reference 8 above.

26. Wennberg, J.E., B.A. Barnes, and M. Zubkoff. Professional uncertainty and the problem of supplier-induced demand. *Soc. Sci. Med.* 1982; 16:811–24.

27. Wennberg, J.E., and A. Gittelsohn. Variations in medical care among small areas. *Sci. Am.* 1982; 246(4):120–34.

28. Hartzema, A.G., and D.B. Christensen. Nonmedical factors associated with the prescribing volume among family practitioners in an HMO. *Med. Care.* 1983; 21:990–1000.

29. See reference 18 above.

30. See reference 6 above.

31. Melmon, K.L., and T.F. Blaschke. The undereducated physician's therapeutic decisions. *N. Engl. J. Med.* 1983; 308:1473–74.

32. See reference 8 above.

33. Fuchs, V.R., and J.P. Newhouse. National Bureau of Economic Research Conference on the Economics of Physician and Patient Behavior: The conference and unresolved problems. *J. Hum. Resour.* 1978; 13(suppl):1–18.

34. See reference 8 above.

35. Eddy, D.M. Variations in physician practice: The role of uncertainty. *Health Aff.* 1984; 3:74–89.

36. Luft, H.S. Variations in clinical practice patterns. *Arch. Intern. Med.* 1983; 143:1861–62.

37. Pineault, R. The effect of medical training factors on physician utilization behavior. *Med. Care.* 1977; 15:51–67.

38. Avorn, J., M. Chen, and R. Hartley. Scientific versus commercial sources of influence on the prescribing behavior of physicians. *Am. J. Med.* 1982; 73:4–8.

39. Avorn, J., and S.B. Soumerai. Improving drug-therapy decisions through educational outreach: A randomized controlled trial of academically based 'detailing.' *N. Engl. J. Med.* 1983; 308:1457–63.

40. Avorn, J., and S.B. Soumerai. A new approach to reducing suboptimal drug use. *J.A.M.A.* 1983; 250:1752–53.

41. See reference 26 above.

42. See reference 27 above.

43. Wennberg, J.E., and A. Gittelsohn. Small area variations in health care delivery. *Science.* 1973; 182:1102–8.

44. Wennberg, J.E., and A. Gittelsohn. Health care delivery in Maine: I. Patterns of use of common surgical procedures. *J. Maine Med. Assoc.* 1975; 66:123–30, 149.

45. Wennberg, J.E., L. Blowers, R. Parker, and A.M. Gittelsohn. Changes in tonsillectomy rates associated with feedback and review. *Pediatrics.* 1977; 59:821–26.

46. Connell, F.A., R.W. Day, and J.P. LoGerfo. Hospitalization of Medicaid children: Analysis of small area variations in admission rates. *Am. J. Public Health.* 1981; 71:606–13.

47. Dietrich, A.J., and H. Goldberg. Preventive content of adult primary care: Do generalists and subspecialists differ? *Am. J. Public Health.* 1984; 74:223–27.

48. Wennberg, J.E. On patient need, equity, supplier-induced demand and the need to assess the outcome of common medical practices. *Med. Care.* 1985; 23:512–20.

49. Bloor, M. Bishop Berkeley and the adenotonsillectomy enigma: An exploration of variation in the social construction of medical disposals. *Sociology.* 1976; 10:43–61.

50. Bloor, M.J., G.A. Venters, and M.L. Samphier. Geographical variation in the incidence of operations on the tonsils and adenoids. An epidemiological and sociological investigation. Part I. *J. Laryngol. Otol.* 1978; 92:791–801.

51. Bloor, M.J., G.A. Venters, and M.L. Samphier. Geographical variation in the incidence of operations on the tonsils and adenoids. An epidemiological and sociological investigation. Part II. *J. Laryngol. Otol.* 1978; 92:883–95.

52. See reference 49 above.

53. Rich, E.C., T.W. Crowson, and D.P. Connelly. Evidence for an informal clinical policy resulting in high use of a very-low-yield test. *Am. J. Med.* 1985; 79:577–82.

54. See reference 48 above.

55. Read, J.L., R.S. Stern, L.A. Thibodeau, D.E. Geer, Jr., and H. Klapholz. Variation in antenatal testing over time and between clinic settings. *J.A.M.A.* 1983; 249:1605–9.

56. See reference 48 above.

57. Eisenberg, J.M. Physician utilization: The state of research about physicians' practice patterns. *Med. Care.* 1985; 23:461–83.

58. See reference 38 above.

59. See reference 18 above.

60. Coleman, J.S., E. Katz, and H. Menzel. *Medical Innovation: A Diffusion Study.* New York: Bobbs-Merrill, 1966.

61. Coleman, J., H. Menzel, and E. Katz. Social process in physicians' adoption of a new drug. *J. Chronic Dis.* 1959; 9:1–9.

62. See reference 38 above.

63. Elstein, A.S., M.M. Holmes, M.M. Ravitch, D.R. Romer, G.B. Holzman, and M.L. Rothert. Medical decisions in perspective: Applied research in cognitive psychology. *Perspect. Biol. Med.* 1983; 16:486–501.

64. Hlatky, M.A., K.L. Lee, E.H. Botvinick, and B.H. Brundage. Diagnostic test use in different practice settings: A controlled comparison. *Arch. Intern. Med.* 1983; 143:1886–89.

65. Cebul, R.D., L.H. Beck, J.G. Carroll, et al. A course in clinical decision making adaptable to different audiences. *Med. Decis. Making.* 1984; 4:285–96.

66. Cebul, R.D. "A look at the chief complaints" revisited. *Med. Decis. Making.* 1984; 4:271–83.

67. Abrams, H.L. The 'overutilization' of x-rays. *N. Engl. J. Med.* 1979; 300:1213–16.

68. Schroeder, S.A. Variations in physician practice patterns: A review of medical cost implications. In Carols, E.J., D. Neuhauser, and W.B. Stason, eds. *The Physician and Cost Control.* Cambridge, Mass.: Oelgeschlager, Gunn & Hain, 1980.

69. See reference 8 above.

70. Pauly, M.V., and M.A. Satterthwaite. The pricing of primary care physicians services: A test of the role of consumer information. In *The Target Income Hypothesis and Related Issues in Health Manpower.* Washington, D.C.: Bureau of Health Manpower, Department of Health, Education and Welfare, 1980; 26–36. DHEW publication no. (HRA) 80–27.

71. See reference 38 above.

72. Hadsall, R.S., R.A. Freeman, and G.J. Norwood. Factors related to the prescribing of selected psychotropic drugs by primary care physicians. *Soc. Sci. Med.* 1982; 16:1747–56.

73. Hall, D. Prescribing as social exchange. In Mapes, R., ed. *Prescribing Practice and Drug Usage.* London: Croom Helm, 1980; 39–57.

74. Vayda, E., and W.R. Mindell. Variations in operative rates: What do they mean? *Surg. Clin. North Am.* 1982; 62:627–39.

75. Roos, N.P. Hysterectomy: Variation in rates across small areas and across physicians' practices. *Am. J. Public Health*. 1984; 74:327–35.

76. Rothert, M.L., D.R. Rovner, A.S. Elstein, G.B. Holzman, M.M. Holmes, and M.M. Ravitch. Differences in medical referral decisions for obesity among family practitioners, general internists, and gynecologists. *Med. Care*. 1984; 22:42–55.

77. Marton, K.I., H.C. Sox, J. Alexander, and C.E. Duisenberg. Attitudes of patients toward diagnostic tests: The case of the upper gastrointestinal series roentgenogram. *Med. Decis. Making*. 1982; 2:439–48.

78. Marton, K.I., H.C. Sox, Jr., J. Wasson, and C.E. Duisenberg. The clinical value of the upper gastrointestinal tract roentgenogram series. *Arch. Intern. Med*. 1980; 140:191–95.

79. See reference 78 above.

80. See reference 76 above.

81. Hulka, B., and J. Wheat. Patterns of utilization: The patient perspective. *Med. Care*. 1985; 23:438–60.

82. Mushlin, A.I., and F.A. Appel. Extramedical factors in the decision to hospitalize medical patients. *Am. J. Public Health*. 1976; 66:170–72.

83. See reference 21 above.

84. Hornbrook, M.C., and M.G. Goldfarb. A partial test of a hospital behavioral model. *Soc. Sci. Med*. 1983; 17:667–80.

85. Uhlmann, R.F., T.S. Inui, and W.B. Carter. Patient requests and expectations. *Med. Care*. 1984; 22:681–85.

86. See reference 85 above.

87. Williams, S.V., J.M. Eisenberg, L.A. Pascale, and D.S. Kitz. Physicians' perceptions about unnecessary diagnostic testing. *Inquiry*. 1982; 19:363–70.

88. Munch, P. Economic incentives to order lab tests: Theory and evidence. In Hough, D.E., and G.I. Misek, eds. *Socioeconomic Issues of Health*. Chicago: American Medical Assoc., 1980; 59–83.

89. Garg, M.L., W.A. Gliebe, and M.B. Elkhatib. The extent of defensive medicine: Some empirical evidence. *Leg. Aspects Med. Practice*. 1978; 6:25–29.

90. Lusted, L. *A Study of the Efficacy of Diagnostic Radiologic Procedures: Final Report to the National Center for Health Services Research, Rockville, Md., 31 May 1977*. Rockville, Md.: National Center for Health Services Research, 1977.

91. Wertman, B.G., S.V. Sostrin, Z. Pavlova, and G.D. Lundberg. Why do physicians order laboratory tests? A study of laboratory test request and use patterns. *J.A.M.A*. 1980; 243:2080–82.

92. Hirsh, H.L., and T.S. Dickey. Defensive medicine as a basis for malpractice liability. *Trans. Stud. Coll. Physicians Phila*. 1983; 5:98–107.

93. Duke Law Project. The medical malpractice threat: A study of defensive medicine. *Duke Law J*. 1971; 5:939–93.

94. Hershey, N. The defensive practice of medicine: Myth or reality. *Milbank Mem. Fund Q*. 1972; 50:69–98.

95. Hayes, L.F. Defensive medicine: The incorrect solution. *Mich. Med.* 1977; 76:267–68.

96. Special Task Force on Professional Liability and Insurance. *Professional Liability in the 80's.* Chicago: American Medical Assoc., October 1984.

97. Upstate surgeons curb practices to offset soaring insurance fees. *New York Times.* 30 May 1985:B8.

98. See reference 97 above.

99. See reference 2 above.

100. Eisenberg, J.M. Sociological influences on decision making by clinicians. *Ann. Intern. Med.* 1979; 90:957–64.

101. See reference 17 above.

102. See reference 28 above.

103. Greenwald, H.P., M.L. Peterson, L.P. Garrison, et al. Interspecialty variation in office-based care. *Med. Care.* 1984; 22:14–29.

104. See reference 17 above.

105. See reference 103 above.

106. Hooper, E.M., L.M. Comstock, J.M. Goodwin, and J.S. Goodwin. Patient characteristics that influence physician behavior. *Med. Care.* 1982; 20:630–38.

107. See reference 17 above.

108. Penchansky, R., and D. Fox. Frequency of referral and patient characteristics in group practice. *Med. Care.* 1980; 8:368–85.

109. See reference 100 above.

110. Rose, H., and B. Abel-Smith. *Doctors, Patients, and Pathology.* London: G. Bell and Sons, 1972. Occasional papers on Social Administration, No. 49.

111. Hardwick, D.F., P. Vertinsky, R.T. Barth, V.F. Mitchell, M. Bernstein, and I. Vertinsky. Clinical styles and motivation: A study of laboratory test use. *Med. Care.* 1975; 13:397–408.

4

The Physician as
Guarantor of Social Good

The previous two chapters describe the multiplicity of interacting factors that influence physicians' provision and use of medical services. They demonstrate that much of the variation in medical practice is due to physicians' attempts to satisfy their personal desires and simultaneously to serve as their patients' agents.

Physicians seem to be most comfortable when they can consider only the welfare of their patients and themselves as the principal issues in medical care decisions (although they may claim to consider only the patient's benefit). While physicians may also be willing to weigh the effect of their decisions on the patient's family, they are generally less comfortable contemplating the impact of their decisions on the rest of society. They are generally unwilling to consider the effect of their individual decisions on the overall cost of medical care or the consumption of limited resources (be they beds, scarce drugs, or dollars). In fact, many doctors believe that these broader considerations have no place in an ethical physician's decision making.

Physicians seem to have greater ease dealing with the allocation of resources that is implicit in decisions that are removed from the individual patient, such as concerns of public hygiene, the communicability of infections, or construction of medical facilities. While these issues still fall within the medical framework, the goal of overall societal benefit is more easily accepted as a factor to be weighed in these decisions because of their clear separation from the doctor-patient relationship.

Although these constraints of society's limited resources have received less attention by physicians in their usual decisions about the care of individual patients than have some of the factors described in the preceding chapters, a decade ago many of these issues did come uncomfortably close to the level of medical decision making. When physicians were faced with limited capacity for renal dialysis, they had to decide whether to use society's limited resources for dialysis on one patient or another. In the end, physicians welcomed the introduction of Medicare coverage for patients with endstage renal disease, in large part because it relieved them of the dilemma of allocating scarce resources among patients [1].

Today, as those who pay the bill for medical care ask ever more probing questions about its cost, physicians are less able to avoid the issue of cost, even in the care of individual patients. Those who pay seem to be somewhat more willing to ask more than just whether a medical intervention's benefit outweighs its risk. They are beginning to ask whether its benefit justifies its cost and whether it is the most cost-effective way to use limited financial resources for medical care.

For the physician protected by the reimbursement systems of traditional fee-for-service practice, the questions of cost benefit and cost effectiveness can still be asked in the abstract, since resources are not often actually limited in the care of individual patients. However, hospital administrators will remind these physicians that prospective payment by diagnosis related group (DRG) limits the hospital's ability to provide services. For the physician practicing in a prepaid, capitated plan such as a health maintenance organization, the question takes on more reality. There really is a fixed amount of money for the prepaid plan's enrollees, and the plan's physicians want to provide the highest quality care they can within those constraints. Anticipating this conflict for the individual physician who may be tempted to withhold an expensive service that offers a small but real clinical contribution to one patient so that the resources can be used to provide substantial benefit to another, Aaron and Schwartz have predicted that American physicians will build into their norms of good practice a sense of the relation between the costs of care and the value of the benefits from it [2].

Economists have described the "moral hazard" for physicians acting as the individual patient's agent and demanding optimal quality care for the individual, especially when these patients are protected from out-of-pocket expenses by a third-party payer. This dilemma is most vexing when the use of scarce resources may be profitable for the doctor and potentially beneficial for the patient but inefficient in terms of all patients [3].

On the other hand, even if individual physicians do recognize that the use of some medical care provides small but positive benefits to them and their patients but means fewer resources for others, why should this knowledge induce any physician to change his or her behavior? After all, whether the individual physician prescribes what he or she thinks will maximize benefit to the patient or avoids doing so because of the social cost, the overall level of medical care use generally will not be perceptibly affected. There will not be enough money saved or spent on the individual patient to make much difference in overall medical care spending.

This dilemma is related to the "prisoner's dilemma" in game theory [4]. In the prisoner's dilemma, one must decide between accepting an equitable distribution of resources (or risk) versus taking more than one's own share and leaving less for others. The decision to take only one's own fair share is complicated by the knowledge that others may decide to play by different, more selfish, rules and take more than their share. Thus, the decision to accept one's share carries with it the risk that less than one's share may be available if others are more selfish.

Furthermore, according to traditional laissez-faire principles (à la Adam Smith), behavior compatible with individual physicians' and patients' interests would be preferred. If each of us acts in our own interest, this philosophy suggests, then it will be as if we were all guided by an invisible hand to promote the public interest.

Therefore, many would propose that it is inappropriate for the physician to accept less than optimal care for individual patients. To accept less in order to leave resources for others who are of equal need has been deemed by some to be unethical behavior. Jonsen, Siegler, and Winsdale, writing in *Clinical Ethics* [5], suggest that the physician is accountable to the patient and not the public. They imply that decision making about individual patients should be made without regard to societal constraints.

A rebuttal to the invisible hand argument can be found in a scenario first described in 1833 by a mathematical amateur named William Forster Lloyd. Hardin has recounted this scenario and entitled it "the tragedy of the commons" [6]. It takes place in a common pasture that is used by a number of herdsmen. As a rational being, each herdsman seeks to maximize his personal gain. He asks himself, "What is the value to me of adding another animal to my herd?" He concludes that the only sensible course is to add another animal, and he does so. But so do all the other herdsmen, and soon thereafter, each adds another animal, followed by even more. The commons becomes overcrowded with animals and there is insufficient grass for grazing. As Hardin describes the dilemma, each man is locked into a system that compels him to increase his herd without limit, in a world that is limited. Each pursues his own best interest in a society that believes in the freedom of the commons, but freedom of the commons brings ruin to all [7].

Somers first drew a parallel from the "tragedy of the commons" to health care several years ago [8], and the analogy is all the more fitting today. As the resources available for medical services are increasingly limited, the dilemma of the individual practitioner will become even more important. As the individual responsible for optimizing the patient's health, the physician would like to be able to use resources as if they were unlimited except by the patient's own resources and values. However, as a responsible member of society, the physician will want to strive for efficiency in the use of medical services. This goal of equity and efficiency suggests that the marginal yield for society should be the same for all medical services in order to ensure efficient allocation of resources. Of course, this allocation will depend on how society defines its values and, therefore, its utilities for medical services, their cost, and their outcomes.

Unfortunately, there are fewer descriptive data than normative exposition about these decisions, so little empirical information is known about how this concern for social good does or will influence medical decision making. The willingness and ability of physicians to address this ethical dilemma vary and may explain some of the variation in medical practice when other variables such as case mix and patient or physician characteristics are controlled.

The decision between spending money on prevention or the treatment of disease typifies the ethical dilemma of how to allocate scarce resources. Even though prevention might save more lives or offer more health for the money spent, it is often given a lower priority than treatment. Why? Menzel, in his book *Medical Costs, Moral Choices*, suggests that treatment may be preferred because in treatment we are helping known, identifiable individuals [9]. "To many," Menzel writes, "it seems morally more important to help identifiable individuals than to do what we perceive will only statistically avert some harm to people whose identity we do not yet know." By choosing treatment over prevention, we are not really avoiding the allocation or rationing of medical care; we have already sacrificed those whose diseases could have been prevented to treat those already afflicted. The doctor is making the decision (or has been encouraged to make it by the third-party payer which refuses to pay for preventive services). Instead of dealing with the dilemma, the physician ignores it.

Individual practicing physicians are perplexed by the demand that they be medical double agents, at once serving their patients and society. This dilemma was the topic of a pair of special articles in *The New England Journal of Medicine* in 1975, one by the dean of the Harvard School of

Public Health [10] and the other by a Harvard law professor [11]. The dean, Howard Hiatt, stated his belief that we can no longer afford the luxury of the principle that one should do everything possible for the individual patient. "We risk reaching a point," he wrote, "where marginal gains to individuals threaten the welfare of the whole," invoking the spirit of the tragedy of the commons. On the other hand, Hiatt sympathized with the unenviable role into which his philosophy of efficiency casts the individual practitioner. He asserted that to ask the physician to withhold care from a patient is not "fair," but he hedged by adding that within the limits available, "the physician . . . must do all that is permitted on behalf of his patient."

The law professor, Charles Fried, took a strikingly different position: "The physician who withholds care that is in his power to give because he judges it is wasteful to provide it to a particular person breaks faith with his patient." Fried argued that people have certain basic rights that go beyond the right to have allocated to them their just share of society's resources. He contended that the individual physician should not be asked to serve as the agent of an efficient health care delivery system.

Although Fried's treatise is an elegant defense of individual liberties, it seems to have been written in isolation from the reality of limited resources. The author either ignored or disagreed with John Donne's principle that "no man is an island." His essay cursed the darkness, but threw no light on the problem of how individual physicians can participate in efforts to contain what many consider to be runaway medical care costs without depriving their own patients of valuable care.

The easiest answer is to eliminate medical care that does not contribute to improved health. This solution suggests that more epidemiologic, economic, and technologic assessment research will provide the information that is needed to avoid "flat of the curve medicine," in which no additional benefits are gained by additional dollars spent. However, the doctor's dilemma would remain when benefits do exist but are small and costs high, especially when people would argue about the value of the benefits. For example, what about the widely recognized high cost of care in the last year of life? Who are the rest of us to judge how valuable that last year is to the patient and family? What about a very expensive diagnostic test that may make a real, but tiny, contribution to a patient's care? While few would argue against reducing medical care costs by eliminating services that contribute nothing to health, heated debate can be evoked by proposals that cost and quality are outcomes of medical care that must be traded off, one against the other.

One solution is to make the decision for the doctors. It is fashionable today for hospitals to establish ethics committees to help make some of these difficult decisions. Some have suggested that these review committees are especially important when the doctor is an employee of the hospital or has a financial interest in the hospital. Whereas ethics committees may prove to be helpful in the difficult, dramatic, life-and-death situations when enough time is available for consultants to be assembled, they are unlikely to help with most medical decisions. Should the expensive test with little but something to add to patient care be ordered? Should an expensive antibiotic that is a little more effective than a much cheaper one be prescribed? There is a multitude of day-to-day decisions in medical practice in which patients' clinical benefit, doctors' economic benefit, and a variety of other factors—in addition to saving the commons for future herdsmen and grazing animals—need to be weighed.

The proposal of medical ethicists Jonsen, Siegler, and Winsdale to let policy makers and program administrators decide on how to ration care is as quixotic as the idea of letting hospital ethics committee do it [12]. Each might work for dramatic and major decisions that involve great cost or great potential clinical benefit. However, neither the committee nor the bureaucrat will be able to guide the physician in most day-to-day clinical decisions, where the bulk of health care expenditures are triggered. While clinically relevant epidemiologic, economic, and decision-analytic research may provide data and conceptual frameworks for the decisions, the dilemma will remain.

The burden still belongs to the doctors, to be shared with the patient. Each can be asked to understand and operate within the limits society has placed on medical care. Although it may not be necessary to go to the extreme that some have proposed— that doctors must inform patients whenever cost is a factor in their medical decisions [13]—the patient should be party to this aspect, as well as others, of medical decision making.

Implicit in this discussion of the moral dilemma of the physician spending large amounts of money for small benefits to an individual patient is the assumption that the costs will be picked up by some third party to the doctor-patient relationship. When substantial costs are not covered by insurance, the government, or some other payer, the patient may bear the costs out of pocket. In this event, it is not only reasonable to share decision making with the patient; it would be unethical not to do so, to preclude the patient from a commitment of his own money.

Perhaps the commons should be expanded. Perhaps the resources available to physicians should be increased so that fewer dilemmas occur about whether limited resources should be spent for a small improvement in health for an individual patient. Perhaps we should spend more on medical care, not less; this is an option to be decided at the societal level.

Political and social decisions about the allocation of society's resources will be made, and it is the doctors' responsibility to have an active role in their making, just as it is their responsibility to use the available resources as effectively as possible at the clinical level.

This book is intended to be a review and analysis of the evidence about how doctors respond to the various pressures on their decision making. It is not intended to prescribe how they should respond. It is about descriptive decision-making research more than about normative decision making. Nonetheless, the problem of the medical commons, the tension between what is best for the individual (doctor or patient) and what is best for society, is too important to overlook. Little empirical research is available about how doctors respond to this problem—the new doctor's dilemma—and how they balance their interpersonal and societal responsibilities. Several philosophical paradigms have been put forth—ranging from proposals that the limits of societal resources be ignored to suggestions that physicians apply cost-effectiveness analysis at the bedside. How practitioners respond to the limited resources available to their practices will provide insights into the philosophy that they adopt.

These chapters have probed the practice of medicine to investigate physicians' practices and to study the factors that influence them. If these insights into the forces that shape medical decision making help to explain some of the variation in clinical practice patterns, then investigation of the effectiveness of efforts to change physicians' practices may elucidate further why doctors practice the way they do.

References

1. Eisenberg, J.M. Sociological influences on decision making by clinicians. *Ann. Intern. Med.* 1979; 90:957–64.

2. Aaron, H.J., and W.B. Schwartz. *The Painful Prescription: Rationing Hospital Care.* Washington, D.C: The Brookings Institution, 1984; 127–28.

3. Pauly, M.V. *Doctors and Their Workshops.* Chicago: National Bureau of Economic Research, The University of Chicago Press, 1980.

4. I am grateful to Mark Pauly for offering this perspective on the prisoner's dilemma.

5. Jonsen, A.R., M. Siegler, and W.J. Winsdale. *Clinical Ethics.* New York: MacMillan Publishing Co., Inc., 1982; 142, 157–59.

6. Hardin, G. The tragedy of the commons. *Science.* 1968; 162:1243–48.

7. See reference 4 above.

8. Somers, A.R. *Health Care in Transition.* Chicago: Hospital Research and Educational Trust, 1971; 153–57.

9. Menzel, P.T. *Medical Costs, Moral Choices: A Philosophy of Health Care Economics in America.* New Haven, Conn.: Yale University Press, 1983.

10. Hiatt, H.H. Protecting the medical commons: Who is responsible? *N. Engl. J. Med.* 1975; 293:235–41.

11. Fried, C. Rights and health care: Beyond equity and efficiency. *N. Engl. J. Med.* 1975; 293:241–45.

12. See reference 5 above.

13. Mahler, D.M., R.M. Veath, and V.W. Sidel. Ethical issues in informed consent: Research in medical cost containment. *J.A.M.A.* 1982; 247:481–85.

Part II

Changing Physicians' Practice Patterns

The unexplained variation in practice styles among physicians, hospitals, and regions suggests that some medical care may be inappropriate. Indeed, when explicit criteria have been applied to medical practice, instances of both overutilization and underutilization have been found. Even when differences in patients' preferences, case mix, and severity of disease have been considered, there are potential improvements in both the cost and quality of care that might result from changes in the practice habits of some physicians. In some instances, the challenge is to convince clinicians with unusual practice styles to adhere to more commonly accepted practice patterns. In other cases, the challenge is to change the practice of average physicians, whose style of practice may be typical of their colleagues, but who may deviate from an optimal pattern as defined by expert opinion or scientific evidence. Whether the mission is to change the practice style of the aberrant physician or to move the modal practice patterns of the profession, the task of changing physician behavior is a challenging one.

5

General Principles:
A Brief Overview

Several recent reviews have analyzed efforts to change physicians' practice patterns [1–5]. With increased attention by the medical community to the cost of care, the past few years have witnessed a number of new programs to change physicians' utilization of services. Concern about the quality of care has also motivated efforts to alter physicians' practices. This review places these recent contributions in the context of the previous literature.

The experiences in modifying medical practice provide valuable insights into the factors that influence physician decision making. In the same way that biological studies of the action and effect of drugs reveal information about physiology and pathophysiology, these efforts to alter physicians' use of medical services offer explanations for the reasons that doctors practice the way they do. In a brief review of this literature, it will be useful to emphasize more recent publications and to concentrate on the way that this literature reveals basic insights into the determinants of physician practice patterns.

Previous chapters have made the point that the factors that influence physicians' use of medical services are complex. They include personal considerations of the physician, such as the aspiration for income, the enjoyment of a satisfying practice, and the desire for approval from peers. Characteristics of the patient and the clinical encounter are also influential, such as consideration of the patient's economic well-being, maintenance or improvement of the patient's health, and understanding of the patient's perceived values and desires. The influence of these desires of the doctor and patient are set in an environment of limited resources, where each physician's use of services for each patient has an impact on society's expenditure for medical care and, ultimately (but indirectly), society's ability and willingness to spend additional dollars for health.

Since the reasons for the use of medical services are multiple, it is unlikely that a simplistic approach to changing physicians' practice patterns will work well. However, understanding why doctors practice as they do should help in designing effective programs to change physician behavior, just as the results of these programs provide additional insights into that behavior. Two related approaches to changing behavior that are valuable in changing physicians' practice patterns come from the social sciences: behavior modification and management theory [6–10].

Clues from Behavior Modification

The early work of B.F. Skinner in the experimental analysis of behavior provides interesting insights into the process of changing physicians' practice behavior [11]. Skinner, elaborating on the "law of effect," suggested that both positive and negative stimuli (reinforcers) can be used to alter the frequency of a behavior. He showed that the frequency may be altered by either presenting or withholding the reinforcer contingent on the behavior. Therefore, any of four strategies, presented in figure 5.1, could be used to change behavior [12]. When a favorable stimulus is presented (for example, money) following a desired behavior, that behavior is positively reinforced and is likely to be repeated. However, when the favorable stimulus is withheld, the behavior will be discouraged (the process of extinction). On the other hand, punishment (the presentation of a negative or aversive stimulus) can also stop the behavior, whereas negative reinforcement (withdrawing an aversive stimulus) increases the frequency of the behavior.

Skinnerian behaviorists have enunciated general principles for developing, modifying, and maintaining behavior that are based on manipulation (scheduling) of these positive and aversive reinforcers [13]. In addition to simple punishment, extinction, positive reinforcement, and negative reinforcement, behaviorists use shaping and reinforcement of competing responses to alter the frequency of behaviors. In shaping behavior, one waits for the individuals to demonstrate a movement in the right direction, that is toward the desired behavior (even if it occurs as a random event), and then reinforces it. Having reinforced the behavior, one waits for a closer approximation to the desired behavior and

Figure 5.1   The Skinnerian model of behavior change.

REINFORCEMENT

	OFFERED	WITHHELD
FAVORABLE STIMULUS	Positive Reinforcement ——— Behavior Increases	Extinction ——— Behavior Decreases
NEGATIVE STIMULUS	Punishment ——— Behavior Decreases	Negative Reinforcement ——— Behavior Increases

Source: Adapted from Skinner, B.F., *The Behavior of Organisms.* New York: Appleton-Century, 1938.

reinforces that. By patiently waiting for and reinforcing these "successive approximations," the desired behavior is encouraged and can become a learned behavior pattern. Conversely, one might discourage a certain behavior by reinforcing a competitive behavior, that is, by encouraging an opposite behavior, one that excludes the undesired behavior. Simultaneously, the undesired behavior can be extinguished by not reinforcing it. Short of making an undesirable behavior physically impossible (as in imprisonment), reinforcing a desirable alternative behavior is the most promising way to maintain a modified behavior.

When applied to human activities, these behavior modification theories suggest that first one must search for clues to identify the reinforcers currently maintaining the behavior to be altered; then appropriate reinforcers should be used to condition new behavior. Although punishment may alter behavior drastically, its result is often transient and complicated by emotional side effects, whereas positive reinforcement often maintains a new behavior indefinitely. Continued reinforcement of the new behavior is generally necessary to maintain behavior and avoid regression to the old behavior. Frequent reinforcement is necessary, at least at the beginning, but intermittent reinforcement is often more durable. Individualized instruction (with personal face-to-face contact) seems to be the most successful way to use education as a mechanism of delivering feedback [14]. These lessons of behavior theory, though not dealing with the more cognitive aspects of behavior, offer useful principles in conceptualizing attempts to alter physicians' practice patterns, particularly with regard to the importance of relevant feedback (ideally delivered personally by a respected individual) and the need to reinforce newly learned behaviors.

Ideas from Management Theory

The contributions of management theory also offer valuable insights toward understanding how physician practice patterns can be altered. One pertinent area of management theory is organizational change. Lewin suggested that successful organizational change has three components: unfreezing, changing behavior, and refreezing [15]. To unfreeze established behavior, it is necessary to create a sense of dissatisfaction and to remove external support for the existing behavior patterns. Next, a "change agent" is needed to propose a new way to behave. To be successful, this change agent should be a person who, for whatever reason, has power and influence in the organization. Finally, the behavior is reinforced, perhaps through the internal culture of the organization or through formal rewards and penalties. Like other theories from the management literature, change theory requires the leadership of key persons. For example, the marketing literature emphasizes the role of pacesetters in establishing purchasing patterns [16, 17].

The principle of unfreezing may be an especially important one now, as the traditional incentives for medical practice are changing rapidly. In particular, prepaid practice and prospective payment of hospitals have removed the external financial support for the full-steam-ahead approach to practice. Undoubtedly, the status quo has been upset, dissatisfaction with the current order is being created, and physicians will probably be more amenable to change in the future. Whether the influential change agents will step forward and whether mechanisms can be established to reinforce the new behavior remain to be seen. Nonetheless, the stage is set for substantial change in medical practice patterns.

Another principle of management theory that is valuable in understanding the process of changing physician behavior is derived from contingency theory, which suggests that the best way to change individual behavior is contingent on the type of work the individual does, the nature of the organization, and the type of people involved [18, 19]. For professionals who deal with ambiguity and operate independently, decentralized and participatory decision making is most successful. In contrast, centralized, hierarchial decision making is a more successful strategy if the organization is bureaucratic, the people are not well educated or professional, and the work is routine.

Lessons from Adult Learning Theory

In addition to the lessons from behavior modification and management theory, valuable insights into changing physician behavior can be gained from education theory [20, 21]. Adult learning theory suggests that adults learn what they think they need to know. Therefore, to teach adults, the educator must determine not only where students' deficiencies lie, but also those areas of knowledge that the students want to learn. Alternatively, the educator can try to create this perceived need and desire for knowledge among potential students.

Implications

Considering these lessons of behavior modification, management, and adult learning theory (presented briefly but I hope not too superficially) and keeping in mind the reasons that doctors seem to practice the way they do, we can put into place a program to change physician behavior. The six general ways in which physicians' practices have been altered are education, feedback, participation, administrative changes, incentives, and penalties. These will be discussed more fully in the next two chapters. Although each method has been successful when used alone, the challenge of changing physician behavior, with its complexity and multiple influences, is most likely to be met successfully by a combination of these strategies.

In studying physicians' responses to efforts to change their behavior, it readily becomes apparent that the bulk of the available data relates to physicians' use of ancillary services (for example, laboratory tests, radiographic examinations, and drug prescriptions). What is less clear is whether the use of these ancillary services is a good indicator of doctors' motivations and responses to interventions.

Ancillary services are used in research on practice patterns not necessarily because they are believed to be the best markers of doctors' practices, but because they are concrete services, explicit data are available about them (usually from chart review or claims forms), and they are ordered with enough frequency to allow statistical analysis. Cognitive and interpersonal services are less easily measured. Interestingly, these reasons are also among those that third-party payers give for paying doctors more for these procedures and concrete services than for cognitive services. The payers and the researchers of physicians' practices do not necessarily value these ancillary services more highly than cognitive services; they simply find them easier to measure.

References

1. Grossman, R.M. A review of physician cost-containment strategies for laboratory testing. *Med. Care*. 1983; 21:783–802.

2. Myers, L.P., and S.A. Schroeder. Physician use of services for the hospitalized patient: A review, with implications for cost containment. *Milbank Mem. Fund Q*. 1981; 59:481–507.

3. Eisenberg, J.M. The use of ancillary services: A role for utilization review? *Med. Care*. 1982; 20:849–61.

4. Eisenberg, J.M., and S.V. Williams. Cost containment and changing physicians' practice behavior: Can the fox learn to guard the chicken coop? *J.A.M.A.* 1981; 246:2195–2201.

5. Eisenberg, J.M. Modifying physicians' patterns of laboratory use. In Connelly, D.P., E.S. Benson, M.D. Burke, and D. Fenderson, eds. *Clinical Decisions and Laboratory Use*. Minneapolis: University of Minneapolis Press, 1982; 145–58.

6. See reference 5 above.

7. Skinner, B.F. *The Behavior of Organisms*. New York: Appleton-Century, 1938.

8. Ferster, C.B., and B.F. Skinner. *Schedules of Reinforcement*. New York: Appleton-Century-Crofts, 1957.

9. Sherman, A.R. *Behavior Modification: Theory and Practice*. Monterey, Calif.: Brooks/Cole Pub. Co., 1973.

10. Lewin, K. Group decision and social change. In Newcomb, T.M., and E.L. Hantley, eds. *Readings in Social Psychology*. New York: Holt, Rinehart and Winston, 1958.

11. See reference 7 above.

12. My thanks to Norman Weissman who clarified this behavioral model for me.

13. See reference 8 above.

14. See reference 9 above.

15. See reference 10 above.

16. Coleman, J.S., E. Katz, and H. Menzel. *Medical Innovation: A Diffusion Study*. New York: Bobbs-Merrill, 1966.

17. Coleman, J., H. Menzel, and E. Katz. Social process in physicians' adoption of a new drug. *J. Chronic Dis*. 1959; 9:1–9.

18. See reference 10 above.

19. Lawrence, P.R., and J.W. Lorsch. *Organization and Environment: Managing Differentiation and Integration*. Cambridge, Mass.: Division of Research, Graduate School of Business Administration, Harvard University Press, 1967.

20. Williamson, J.W., D.M. Barr, E. Fee, et al. *Teaching Quality Assurance and Cost Containment in Health Care: A Faculty Guide*. San Francisco: Jossey-Bass, 1982.

21. Williamson, J.W., J.I. Hudson, and M.M. Nevins. *Principles of Quality Assurance and Cost Containment in Health Care.* San Francisco: Jossey-Bass, 1982.

6

Do Education and Feedback Change Doctors' Decisions?

Because physicians who are more knowledgeable and clinically mature ○ use fewer and more appropriate diagnostic tests and other medical services, as the research reviewed in previous chapters suggests, it follows logically that education should improve the use of these services. In this context, the idea of education implies that information or skills will be transferred with the intention of increasing students' understanding of the appropriate use of medical care services and improving their use of the services. Although some authors include feedback about a practitioner's practice patterns as a type of education, doing so confuses the cognitive influence of knowledge itself with the behavioral influence of feedback, which is usually based on norms or implies that a norm exists. Therefore, this chapter attempts to separate more clearly the influence of feedback from that of education.

Will Education Change Doctors' Practices?

Unfortunately, much of the literature on educational interventions to alter physicians' prescription of medical services simply reports planned programs of education with little or no evaluation [1, 2]. At the same time, many of the published evaluations that have critically assessed the effectiveness of education in changing physicians' practice patterns and have used reasonable research methods describe programs that were conducted at academic medical centers. Because practice patterns of trainees clearly differ from those of community practitioners, the degree to which these results can be generalized is limited.

Furthermore, some studies have been done without control groups and simply represent descriptions of utilization patterns before and after an intervention [3–5]. When adequate controls have been included, investigators often have been surprised to find changes in the control practices as well, thus casting doubt on the effect of the transmission of information or skills through education isolated from other influences [6]. For example, one study noted that coincident with an education program the authors had credited with a decrease in the use of skull radiographic examinations, there was a decrease in all radiographic examinations [7]. The authors did not comment on whether this decrease reflected a general decrease in test ordering that was independent of the program or whether the decrease was due to spillover from the education about skull radiography. The absence of adequate controls prevented them from ascertaining the cause.

In addition, many programs have concentrated on only a few services, so it has been difficult to know whether other services were affected, perhaps even experiencing a compensatory increase in utilization [8–10]. Therefore, although the literature on educational programs to alter physicians' practice patterns is large, the methodological limitations of most of these evaluations preclude a strong conclusion that education alone alters physicians' practices.

In addition to these methodological limitations, the evidence that education alone can effectively change physicians' practice patterns is unconvincing because so many of the carefully designed investigations have failed to show any effect of education on utilization [11, 12], even though attitudes of the students may have improved [13]. Others have found limited effects of education. For example, in one study education was less important than simply altering the order form for requesting laboratory tests [14], and in another education was successful in altering the use of old services but not use of new services [15].

Despite these disheartening results, the sheer bulk of the reports about educational attempts to change doctors' practices deserves attention. Some who have reviewed this literature have reached more optimistic conclusions about the effectiveness of education. For example, in one extensive review of continuing medical education, Davis and colleagues identified and assessed 238 articles [16]. Few of the studies satisfied the rigorous criteria for methodological adequacy established by the authors, such as including controls, randomly assigning subjects, assessing educational needs in advance, recording attendance (or compliance with the educational program), minimizing the possibility of simultaneous interventions, and avoiding contamination of the control group. Despite these limitations, the reviewers conclude that continuing medical education can have an effect on the competence and performance of participating physicians. They argue that the inconsistent and often discouraging results from studies of education to change physicians imply only that more rigorous research is needed, not to mention better education. Davis and colleagues point out that education has many approaches and that not all physicians are alike. Their conclusion that work is needed to identify which interventions work for which doctors is consistent with the principles of contingency theory that were reviewed in the previous chapter—the method of change should fit the character of those who are to be changed. Perhaps the answer is best expressed by paraphrasing Harold Begbie's famous statement about the Christian ideal: education has not been tried and found wanting; it has been found to be difficult and left untried.

Others also have not lost faith in the potential of education alone. Soumerai and Avorn, in their excellent and comprehensive review of cost-containment efforts in pharmacotherapy, remind the skeptic that education is not a "unidimensional intervention which is either effective or ineffective" [17]. Their analysis of the large literature on changing doctors' prescription of drugs does indicate that printed drug information materials, when used alone, are not effective. However, they conclude that other educational approaches, such as face-to-face education, may work.

McDonald and colleagues have suggested that the effectiveness of computer reminders and the relative lack of effectiveness of education alone are due to the fact that education can actuate physicians' existing intentions but not alter these intentions [18]. They suggest that when education works, it does so because physician errors are more often due to oversights than ignorance. Others have suggested that education is limited as a strategy for change because it is unusual for the problem in physician practice patterns to be a lack of knowledge per se [19].

Despite these caveats, some well-designed programs of education have succeeded in changing physicians' practice patterns. Both the success of these programs and the failure of others to induce lasting changes in the utilization of medical services offer insights into the practice behavior of physicians. For example, Griner was able to produce lasting change in the use of diagnostic tests at Strong Memorial Hospital in Rochester, New York [20]. Although Griner's program actually included some interventions that cannot be described as educational but were more administrative, other investigators have also shown successful results from education alone.

One popular educational strategy has been to teach physicians about the cost of medical care services. Grossman has described these as cost-awareness programs [21]. This approach has had mixed results. Although Everett and coworkers found that simply educating physicians about the cost of services was not successful [22], most published reports of programs to educate doctors about costs of care describe decreases in utilization of approximately 30 percent, particularly in the use of diagnostic tests [23–29]. In one study, the number of tests decreasing most in response to cost information was for patients who were less acutely ill [30]. The investigators concluded that residents are more conscious of price when there is less risk associated with having less information about the patient. This conclusion is consistent with the role of the physician as the patient's clinical agent, who is seeking to improve health, which was described in chapter 3. Similarly, the effect of price on utilization is consistent with the role of the physician as the patient's economic agent, because one would expect an increase in price to be perceived by the physician as having an adverse effect on the patient's finances.

Another popular educational strategy has been to provide explicit guidelines for the use of services. Although these programs may have some limited effectiveness [31, 32], most reports of their success are anecdotal and descriptive, rather than analytical, and few have been well-designed trials. In general, printed guidelines are not effective interventions. This approach has generally been unsuccessful on utilization of diagnostic tests, drugs, and other services, such as blood transfusions [33, 34].

Many of these cost-consciousness programs have been aimed at students rather than residents or practicing physicians. These programs apparently have been inspired by the hope that, as Wordsworth wrote, "The child is father to the man," and that habits or knowledge acquired in medical school will shape the graduates' practices. Whereas some of these programs seem to have been effective, others have had less success. For example, Williams and associates designed a multi-pronged educational program for medical students that received positive subjective responses from students but had no measurable effect on their attitudes, knowledge, or performance [35]. Unfortunately, most educational programs for students that have been successful have had to settle for indirect measures of effectiveness, because students do not have independent responsibility for patient care and therefore do not exhibit practice patterns that can be measured [36–39].

The organization that has supported much of this medical student teaching on cost containment, the National Fund for Medical Education, has accepted the limitations of previous efforts to use education alone and has confessed that the process is more complicated than first envisioned

[40]. In fact, the Fund has given up on direct instruction to medical students and residents on cost containment but is maintaining its interest in teaching practicing physicians. The Fund's president, John Freymann, has written that more imaginative programs are needed than traditional education [41].

For example, in addition to providing information about medical care costs, some investigators of physician behavior have tested the effect of computer reminders. McDonald and colleagues have found that computer reminders about preventive measures do prevent physicians from overlooking these services [42]. In this case, the education served to increase utilization. Wilson and associates also found that information provided by computers can influence practice [43]. When computer-tabulated information about patients' histories, results of previous diagnostic tests, an outpatient problem list, and a list of known inpatient and outpatient diagnoses were given to physicians, their use of diagnostic tests decreased from an average of 3.2 per visit to 2.7. This decrease in test ordering was accompanied by an average savings per patient on the emergency room bill of $15.

The results of these computer reminder programs point out the important role of uncertainty in medical practice. In the absence of reliable information, physicians will seek additional data, and providing them with guidelines (such as those for preventive measures) may help to reduce ambiguity and uncertainty in physicians' practices. In a similar vein, when physicians were given explicit criteria for the use of antibiotics, the proportion of cases in which antibiotics were used appropriately increased from 52 percent to 78 percent and the proportion of acceptable doses increased from 80 percent to 98 percent [44].

Still another approach to helping doctors is to teach them how to deal with uncertainty rather than to give them more facts. The National Fund for Medical Education has taken this tack in some of the projects it has supported recently. For example, the faculty of Stanford University are assembling a videotaped and computer-based instructional program on decision analysis [45]. Faculty at the University of Pennsylvania have written a book for teachers of medical decision making in order to disseminate these principles more widely [46]. Preliminary reports from a project at the University of Connecticut suggest that this new approach of teaching doctors how to handle the uncertainty of medical decision making may be more successful than previous educational programs. Early data indicate that residents receiving a curriculum on probabilistic reasoning ordered fewer tests than those receiving a cost-control curriculum [47].

The success of educational programs is likely dependent on more than merely the fit between the content of the teaching and its recipient. Another important element is the type of behavior at which the program is aimed. In the prescription of drugs, for example, it appears that physicians are more amenable to efforts to improve the quality of their prescribing to reduce side effects and optimize drug efficacy than they are when cost containment is the goal [48]. Similarly, the success in reducing utilization of one program's simple manual about laboratory testing may have been due to the fact that it was aimed at outpatient testing (even so, the reduction in the actual number of tests ordered did not reach statistical significance) [49]. Because of the intensity of inpatient care and the multitude of forces on the house officer, it is not surprising that testing for hospitalized patients might be more difficult to reduce.

The above studies suggest that the simple transfer of information is sometimes sufficient to alter practice patterns. However, more than simply providing information is usually necessary. The target of the change effort, the type of education, and the characteristics of the recipient are all critical. In addition, the way in which the information is delivered is important in determining the effect of the education, and other programs to alter practice patterns are usually needed in conjuction with education. The following sections deal with these issues.

The Role of Professional Leadership in Education

In reviewing the literature on continuing medical education, Sanazaro has concluded that no single cause of change is necessary or sufficient to produce a desired change in practice patterns [50]. He points out the need for a professional environment that is conducive to learning and changing practice patterns, and he emphasizes the critical importance of commitment to change by professional leadership. His conclusions about continuing medical education are consistent with those of the literature that demonstrate the importance of a doctor's professional environment in determining practice patterns. Instead of trying to attack this environment, successful programs have generally taken advantage of the professional environment.

The results of studies by Stross and colleagues illustrate the important role of clinical leadership in changing practice patterns [51, 52]. In two programs, one to change practice patterns in the care of patients with arthritis and one for patients with chronic lung disease, leading community physicians were recruited as the instruments of change. In both studies, the investigators identified the educationally influential physicians, the ones to whom others turned for advice, at several Michigan hospitals. These physicians returned home after a short course at the University of Michigan, where they had been educated about the pertinent clinical issues. They had not been instructed in methods of changing behavior or methods of teaching. In both cases, substantial changes were seen in the practice patterns at the community hospitals where the physicians practiced, apparently as a result of informal education of peers by these influential physicians.

In the program that altered the management of pulmonary disease, Stross and colleagues found that 90 percent of the contacts between educationally influential physicians and other physicians were initiated by their colleagues about specific patients. Half of these contacts were formal consultations, while the other half were "curbside" consultations. Personal contact, as opposed to written consultation, was important, and two-thirds of the interactions took place at the nursing station. The educationally influential doctors had contact with 69 percent of primary physicians at their hospitals within one year, and their influence seemed to spread beyond the care of patients about whom they had been consulted. Whereas formal continuing education by the clinical leaders may have played a role, this role was secondary to their personal contact with physicians who looked to them for guidance.

Others have also described the critical role of participation by professional leadership in educational programs designed to alter utilization patterns [53, 54]. When the information is transmitted by mail, it is not as successful as when it is communicated personally by these influential physicians [55]. The important effect of respected leaders is consistent with reports about factors that influence practice patterns and demonstrates the way that efforts to change practice behavior provide insights into the reasons for the utilization of services by physicians.

In reviewing how physicians view the process of change in their practices, Geertsma and colleagues also emphasize the key role of professional colleagues [56]. They suggest that about 37 percent of change occurs because of the influence of colleagues and 34 percent is caused by journal articles. They indicate that journal articles convey not only the information reported, but also convey the prestige of the journal itself, of the professional organization that publishes the journal, and of the authors. Only 5 percent of reported change was due to formal continuing education.

The important role of respected professional peers in making education a successful intervention is consistent with the literature about how innovations diffuse, both in medicine and in general. The literature on persuasive communication lists five attributes of successful communication: its source, the channel or medium of presentation, the characteristics of the audience, the message itself, and the setting [57]. Recommendations are usually most readily accepted when they are delivered personally by a respected source. This suggests that, in general, the most potent legitimizing force for influencing medical practice is professional, face-to-face contact. Even group education aimed at changing practice patterns seems to depend on the aura of the teacher [58].

One important way in which drug companies take advantage of this important role of peer influence in marketing their products is by educating the professional leadership about new drugs and new uses for old drugs. Another is by sending representatives to visit the physician, which is especially successful when the same salesman visits physicians several times and develops personal relationships with them [59].

In an effort to use this same principle of personalized education, Avorn and Soumerai found that face-to-face education of physicians by trained pharmacists led to decreased use of the three types of drugs targeted in the study: cerebral vasodilators, oral cephalosporins, and propoxyphene [60]. This personal interaction was a more powerful influence than printed educational materials.

In a similar study from Tennessee, personal visits by pharmacists were more successful than letters in altering physicians' prescribing habits, but visits by physicians were more successful than those by pharmacists. Figure 6.1 presents the attributable reductions in drug prescribing due to teaching by drug educators and by physician counselors according to the number of doctors prescribing, the number of patients receiving prescriptions, and the number of prescriptions written for contraindicated antibiotics and oral cephalosporins [61]. The education program was designed to be nonthreatening, was focused on doctors who seemed to be overprescribing drugs according to a review of third-party payer claims by their patients, and had the support of the important state professional medical societies. Physicians who received the letter changed no more than physicians in the control group did. In fact, only one-third of them even kept the educational material that was mailed. Although pharmacists were not as successful in changing prescribing patterns as physicians were, their professionalism and knowledge were important in accomplishing the significant effect that they did have.

Therefore, both of these research groups found that the pharmacists were successful when using face-to-face education in changing physicians' prescribing habits. The less impressive results for the pharmacists in the Tennessee study may have been due to their only spending one 15-minute period with the physicians, whereas the pharmacists in the Avorn and Soumerai study visited more than once. There was also larger intergroup variability in the Tennessee study [62–64].

The role of attending physicians in influencing the use of laboratory

Figure 6.1   Attributable reductions in drug prescribing due to
teaching by drug educators and physician counselors.
Attributable reductions (difference between percent
change in prescribing in visit region and that in control/
smaller region) in numbers of doctors prescribing,
numbers of patients receiving, and numbers of
prescriptions written for contraindicated antibiotics and
oral cephalosporins. Open bars denote effect of drug
educator; stripped bars that of physician counselors.

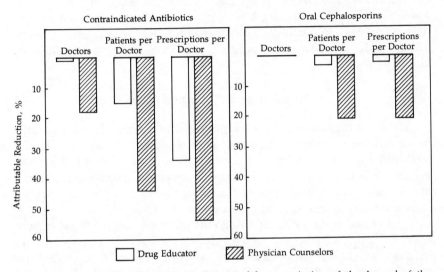

Source: Schaffner and colleagues [61]. Reprinted by permission of the *Journal of the American Medical Association,* 1983; 250:1731. Copyright 1983, American Medical Association.

tests by trainees follows the same principles. Active involvement by faculty in face-to-face teaching of students and residents and the faculty's
stature in the institution are important factors in the success of these
programs at teaching hospitals. Perhaps the frequent resistance of residents to change is related to their faculty's usual lack of enthusiasm for
curtailing the use of diagnostic tests. When faculty were grading students
at one medical school, they did not consider the appropriateness of students' use of general screening tests or tests to investigate unlikely diagnoses in the grades they gave the students. Financial costs, the costs of
false-positive tests leading to further testing, and concern for laboratory
utilization were not considered important enough to weigh inappropriate
usage negatively [65]. This finding suggests that faculty probably tend to

value laboratory test use more on intellectual grounds than on cost-effectiveness grounds [66].

On the other hand, faculty influence sometimes may be taken too far in the opposite direction. In one surgical residency, the department chairman, who was concerned about the overuse of urinalyses in the hospital, told his residents at a conference to take sips of a yellow liquid from urine containers, hoping that it would shock them into reconsidering their use of urinalyses [67]. Although the residents stopped their overuse of the test, they took offense at the method, even though the yellow liquid was not urine. The chairman apologized and admitted, "It was a prank that went awry in the telling but not in what it was supposed to do." This example is a bit Draconian but does exemplify the influence of senior physicians in influencing the practices that their residents and students adopt.

Education and Perceived Need

In addition to the importance of the person who delivers the message and the contribution of face-to-face contact, the physician must perceive a need to change. The transmission of facts alone is insufficient. Stein has written, "When a group of practitioners discover that they need additional facts to deal with a troublesome clinical problem, an episodic learning experience can change clinical performance" [68].

Sanazaro's review of continuing education also supports the importance of creating a perceived need for change among physicians [69]. This principle is fundamental in adult learning theory and helps to explain the importance of uncertainty in influencing utilization patterns. It suggests that if the clinical evidence for a change in practice patterns is clear, physicians will be more likely to respond to simple information. For example, efforts to reduce physicians' prescription of the antibiotic chloramphenicol, a single, simple clinical decision for which preferable alternatives usually exist, have been successful [70]. However, if the situation is more uncertain, as is usually the case in medical care, the physician needs to be convinced that change is desirable, and influential professional leaders are important in creating that perception among other practitioners.

The importance of dissatisfaction with the status quo is also an important principle of change theory in the literature on management and organizational behavior, as was reviewed in chapter 5. Consistent with this strategy, a pilot program was developed to review the use of ancillary services in 25 Massachusetts hospitals [71]. When as many as 30 percent of tests and cardiac services were shown to be inappropriate, the hospitals developed plans for corrective action. Their action, in response to a documented problem, may illustrate the reason that educational efforts to change the use of a single test that has been shown to be overused are more successful than more broadly targeted attempts to alter test use [72, 73].

The importance of physicians' perceptions that change is desirable could be a critical factor in changing their practice patterns as pressure mounts on hospitals and their staffs to contain medical costs. If the introduction of prospective payment by diagnosis related group, increased competition, and greater cost consciousness by third-party payers is perceived by physicians to necessitate that they practice more parsimonious medicine, then it is likely that physicians will be more receptive to educational programs. With such a major change in the economic pressures on physicians, they may soon be ready audiences for programs that teach them to provide quality care efficiently.

Does the Change Persist?

Even when educational programs are successful in changing practice patterns of physicians, the results are often transient. Early reports in the literature on changing physicians' use of diagnostic tests described educational programs that were successful for a short term; physicians returned to their previous behavior when the education was discontinued [74–77]. Figure 6.2 shows the short-lived decrease in the ordering of prothrombin time determinations after a successful educational program [78]. Similar results have been reported more recently, showing that decreased utilization is often short-lived [79], but one study has found persistence of the decreases in inappropriate prescribing [80]. In contrast, distribution of a hospital drug bulletin was effective in altering prescribing patterns for only three weeks and old prescribing patterns soon returned [81]. Another study has claimed to find an effect, albeit modest, of educational programs in medical school that was detectable in the laboratory test ordering of residents several years later [82].

The effect of educational programs, when successful, may be due to the acquisition of new knowledge, but physicians do not necessarily incorporate new information as a result of the education. Changes in attitude may be more critical than information as physicians adopt the values of the educators [83]. One educational program for medical students resulted in the intended change in their attitudes about the use of diagnostic tests, even though no change in knowledge was measurable and their use of tests for simulated cases did not change [84].

In summary, education may succeed in changing physicians' prescription of medical services, but causing this change to occur is not as simple as just providing doctors with information. The perceived needs

Figure 6.2   Return to previous levels of utilization after a briefly
                  successful educational program to reduce use of
                  prothrombin time determinations.

Percentage of patients
having Prothrombin Time

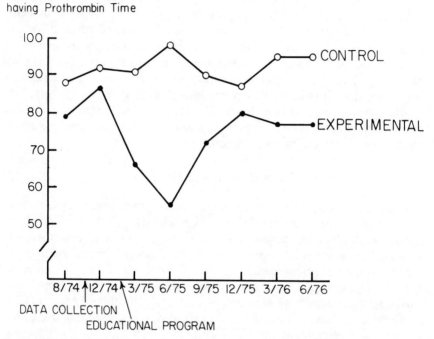

Source: Eisenberg [73]. Reprinted by permission of the *Journal of Medical Education*, 1977;
52:579.

of clinicians must be understood and then met by the educational program. Physicians' attitudes must be considered and perhaps altered. The
active involvement of professional leadership is critical, and personal contact with the educator seems to be most successful. If physicians understand the need for change, then education will be more likely to alter their
practice style. Simple, single clinical actions (for example, the use of a
single drug or test, perhaps especially so in outpatient practice) are probably more amenable to change than are more complex, generic practice
patterns (for example, use of all diagnostic tests), especially when physicians can be convinced by educational methods of the need to change.
In today's era of increasing concern about health care costs, education
about the cost and ways to practice medicine more efficiently is more
likely to achieve some success. However, continued education is probably
necessary to maintain the effect.

A Second Approach: Feedback

Whereas traditional educational methods have attempted to change physician behavior by imparting new knowledge (but with limited success), another group of programs has been designed to change practice patterns by informing physicians about their own behavior. In understanding the factors that influence physicians' practice, it is important to distinguish the effect of this feedback (which has behavioral implications beyond the simple transmission of information) from the effect of conventional education.

The use of feedback to change physicians' practice has been described as an application of "cybernetic control." According to cybernetic theory, the essential means of achieving control over performance of any system is through the use of feedback. By providing feedback, the system can be made to regulate itself [85]. In relating the importance of feedback to medical care, Ende has emphasized the generic importance of feedback in medical education, suggesting that clinical skill, "like ballet, is best learned in front of a mirror" [86]. To improve medical education, Ende suggests that faculty and students work together as allies, that they measure performance against well-defined goals, that the trainees take an active part in the process, and that the feedback be appropriately and accurately descriptive of the trainees' behavior.

Feedback has been applied widely by researchers trying to alter physicians' use of medical services. Performance has been compared with that of peers, statistical standards, both explicit and implicit criteria, and the yield in new diagnoses or successful clinical outcomes. Several reviews have summarized the results of feedback programs, which are usually reported to be successful [87–91]. However, Fineberg and associates have pointed out the possibility that this literature could be biased because of the tendency to publish only the results of successful efforts [92]. This bias is probably especially likely when the evaluator is the same person or team who has designed and carried out the intervention, as is often the case in these programs.

From early studies, such as that of Schroeder and colleagues [93], to more recent programs [94–96], findings have suggested that simply providing performance feedback to physicians might change their use of diagnostic tests. However, the findings are conflicting, because other efforts to distribute feedback with no other intervention (or just in conjunction with education) have not been effective [97–99]. Retrospective drug use reviews that apply one-time feedback of results have generally been ineffective, and results of studies evaluating drug utilization audits followed by group discussions have been difficult to interpret because of methodologic flaws. Despite the numerous occasions over many years in which drug utilization audits have been combined with group educational strategies, not one well-controlled study has been published [100].

Many of the successful programs using feedback to change physicians' practices have suggested that this approach can improve the quality of care as well as reduce its cost. For example, several investigators have described feedback programs that have been aimed at the appropriate use of drugs or transfusions [101–103]. Gehlbach and colleagues have recently reported that computerized feedback increased the use of generic drugs from 21 percent to 58 percent, a significant increase compared with that of a control group [104]. In contrast to their early work [105], this intervention had a lasting effect, with little decay being noted over a 12-month period. There was also spillover of the newly learned behavior to a number of "silent" drugs about which no feedback had been provided.

Is the Medium More Important Than the Message?

While evidence suggests that the simple transmission of performance information to physicians may alter their behavior, feedback is most successful when it is offered face-to-face by a respected member of the medical community, when it is individualized for the physician, and when it represents current, or at least recent, data. Information about practice patterns alone is usually necessary but often not sufficient to change physicians' practice patterns [106]. As is the case with education, the influence of the social structure of practice is critical in modifying physician decision making with the use of feedback [107].

The importance of respected colleagues and the critical role of the social structure of practice help to explain why the most successful programs of performance feedback have involved individuals in positions of clinical leadership. The importance of leadership has been especially evident in efforts to change the test-ordering behavior of housestaff, who practice in hospitals with well-defined hierarchical, social, and professional structures. In fact, Martin and colleagues suggested that the success of their chart audit program at the Brigham and Women's Hospital in Boston was due, at least in part, to the transmission of new attitudes or a value system from the faculty to the residents [108]. In another study, feedback to residents about the cost of diagnostic services that they prescribed was less important than the active involvement by faculty leaders of the housestaff teams [109]. Still another study found that chart review feedback worked better than education or cost audits alone, and that passive teaching of housestaff about costs did not seem to have a meaningful effect; in contrast, active involvement by faculty was consistently successful [110]. Other reports have confirmed the importance of faculty involvement [111, 112].

Individualized personal feedback by a respected clinician has also seemed to be a successful way to change physician practice in community practice settings [113–115]. For example, one community hospital required that when a chart audit detected unnecessary pacemaker implantation, the physician involved had to justify the implantation before a committee of peers [116]. Decreases of more than half were seen in the number of pacemaker implantations. The success of the feedback provided in the often quoted study of tonsillectomy by Wennberg and colleagues [117] probably depended on the active involvement by leaders in the local professional community.

The conclusion that the influence of the professional environment is critical to the success of feedback programs was also shown in a Boston health maintenance organization [118]. Three different interventions were compared in an effort to improve physician performance in colorectal cancer screening. Neither an educational meeting of the staff nor impersonal retrospective feedback of group compliance rates resulted in a significant improvement. However, when monthly feedback included individual physicians' performances ranked with those of their peers (peer comparison feedback), significant improvement occurred and persisted.

Four feedback programs that failed to alter utilization patterns may be the exceptions that prove this rule that active involvement of clinical leadership is critical. Forrest and coworkers placed patients' bills and itemizations directly onto the chart of every patient in a surgery service at a teaching hospital and found no change in utilization patterns [119]. Second, in Australia, Grivell and associates found no effect of peer comparison feedback on the cost and number of laboratory tests [120]. This feedback was done impersonally by the hospital's department of clinical biochemistry and active interpersonal intervention was purposefully avoided in order to eliminate the possibility of peer pressure. Third, Williams and Eisenberg found that feedback to residents about the results of chart audits or the necessity of laboratory testing was not effective in changing practice patterns [121]. This program also did not routinely include personalized face-to-face feedback by faculty clinicians. Fourth, Schroeder and colleagues observed no significant reductions in the first year of their feedback and education program to reduce inpatient costs [122]. In the second year, they involved some attending physicians as well as housestaff and found that the interventions had a slightly greater effect. However, they concluded that one reason for the lack of a substantial effect of their program in either year was their failure to involve clinical leadership in the hospital, particularly the larger group of attending physicians who might have been less supportive of cost containment. These

four unsuccessful programs shared a characteristic: they all provided feedback in a rather impersonal way, without recruiting the active involvement of clinical leadership in personally delivering the feedback.

A more recent report from Stanford [123] suggests that the failure
of feedback in these programs may have been due to another common
problem, the difficulty of changing use of diagnostic tests for inpatients.
The inpatient service, with its large number of severely ill patients and
usually overtired residents (who are bombarded with so much information that it could amount to sensory overload), may be so conducive to
laboratory overuse that it is especially difficult to change.

The Stanford investigators compared the effect of two interventions
designed to change residents' use of outpatient diagnostic tests: an educational manual and feedback about the residents' test ordering. Both
interventions consisted almost solely of printed material that required
little personal input by the instructor. In this remarkably well-designed
study, Marton and colleagues found that the average charge for diagnostic
tests fell from about $31 per visit to between $21 and $23 for three groups:
the residents given the manual, residents given feedback, and residents
given both. The charges for laboratory tests over time are shown in figure
6.3. Although the number of tests ordered changed in the same direction,
the reduction did not quite reach statistical significance. When case mix
was controlled, the results were somewhat different, with the feedback
group changing very little, but the manual and manual-plus-feedback
groups changing markedly. The researchers did not note a diminution in
the residents' response during three months of follow-up, but they admitted their uncertainty about how long the effect would last. Interestingly, patients cared for by residents in the manual-plus-feedback group
were somewhat more likely to indicate that their physician had ordered
too few laboratory tests. (In chapter 3, these investigators were the ones
who identified patient demand as an important factor in doctors' decisions to order upper gastrointestinal series.)

The Stanford researchers concluded that, for outpatient diagnostic
tests, a combination of approaches is more likely to be successful than a
single intervention. Although they did not include personalized feedback
in their intervention, they also did not comment on whether residents
knew that these researchers (who were respected, active clinical faculty)
had written the manual and were organizing the feedback program.

Therefore, for both educational and feedback programs, success in
altering practice patterns could be due to the charisma or the social and
professional influence of the respected clinician who delivers the education or feedback. It is the exceptional feedback program that works when
the source of the feedback is unknown or not respected by the physicians
who are being targeted. In successful feedback programs, it may be that

Figure 6.3   Modify test-ordering behavior in an outpatient medical clinic. Charges for laboratory tests over time. (Mean laboratory charges per patient per visit are compared for four house staff groups during control period and intervention period. Circles indicate control group; squares, manual group; triangles, feedback group; diamonds, manual-plus-feedback group; open figures, no intervention; and closed figures, intervention was underway).

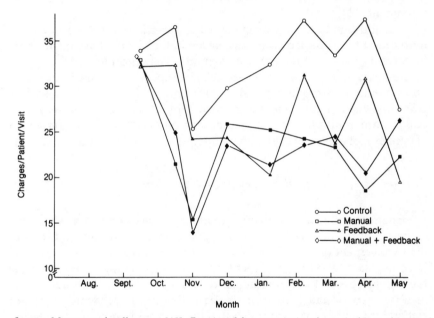

CHARGES FOR TESTS

Source: Marton and colleagues [49]. Reprinted by permission from *Archives of Internal Medicine,* 1985; 145:818.

the fund of knowledge of the practitioners is unchanged. For example, the results of one program, which found reductions in the use of six out of seven types of diagnostic tests after resident-faculty interaction occurred in the review of charts, suggest that change could be due to the effect of the interaction on attitudes or styles of practice rather than on knowledge [124]. In this study, no improvement was seen on examination of the residents' knowledge about the value of diagnostic tests, despite their improved performance.

The importance of the active involvement of clinical leadership in feedback programs may help to explain the mixed success of Professional Standards Review Organizations (PSRO). The PSRO groups that were considered successful seemed to be characterized by aggressiveness (as indicated by the use of surgical necessity review programs) and by contact between doctors (as indicated by the physician density of the region) [125]. Even when physicians are not directly involved, the judgemental, flexible use of explicit clinical criteria established by local experts in timely utilization review is correlated with success [126, 127]. As Sanazaro has suggested, changing physician behavior is most successful when it is done with "regular, timely, salient, individualized feedback on performance compared with explicit standards" in a conducive professional environment [128].

In addition to the advantage of using personalized face-to-face communication by respected clinicians, several other factors have been found important in successful feedback programs. They include visible support of authority figures (which is especially important in residencies and other hierarchical organizations), attention to quality of care as well as cost, information that will be perceived by clinicians to be useful in patient care, multiple approaches that are mutually reinforcing, provision of evidence of excessive utilization, and frequency of feedback [129].

Is the Bang Worth the Buck?

Although performance feedback can alter physician behavior when it is delivered optimally, feedback programs are time consuming and require the involvement of the leaders of the professional community (who often have the least time to spare). Schroeder and associates, in reporting the modest success of their program of combined lectures, chart audit, and feedback (an overall 3 percent decrease in utilization, which was not statistically significant), concluded that the declines in ordering of selected services were not sufficient to suggest a significant impact [130]. Out of an average laboratory bill of $3,000, their program was responsible for savings of $65. Because of the intensity of the intervention, its cost was substantial, averaging $62 per patient (82 percent of which was labor costs) and nullifying the small savings. The successful feedback program at the Brigham and Women's Hospital was also expensive, costing $15,000 for six chart review sessions with all first-year residents [131].

The high cost of these programs helps explain why estimates of the net savings from PSRO programs were controversial. Although some PSRO groups were successful in decreasing the number of hospital days, their benefit-to-cost ratio was estimated to be between 1.16 and 1.65, with substantial variation among programs [132]. The former director of the federal agency responsible for PSRO programs, defending these programs, has pointed out the limitations of these analyses, which were conducted early in the life of the PSROs and did not consider the program's other goals, such as assurance of quality of care [133].

Even with the mixed results of feedback programs, the strength of the evidence that feedback can be a cost-effective way of reducing utilization is limited by faults in the research design of many of the evaluations. The design of these research studies has often been insufficient to determine whether the changes in practice patterns were due to the program or to some other factor. For example, Roberts and colleagues have illustrated the potential in poorly controlled evaluations for concurrent activities at the hospital to cause changes in utilization that would be mistakenly interpreted as a result of the feedback program [134]. They showed that simultaneous administrative changes made it difficult to evaluate the independent effect of feedback. Similarly, Sherman has shown that the mere announcement of an audit program can be associated with changes in behavior, the so-called sentinel effect (which causes change by letting individuals know that they are being monitored and that punishment might be forthcoming) [135]. The sentinel effect is a special case of the well-known Hawthorne effect. In another study, utilization rates had already begun to drop before the audit program was started, which would not have been detected by a simple research design examining before-and-after effects [136].

As new methods of changing physician behavior are developed, the relationship between the cost of these programs and their financial benefit deserves more attention. More efficient methods need to be developed, such as retrospective review [137] and the use of computerized data bases, that will provide less expensive information about utilization, as well as case mix, than can be obtained through labor-intensive chart reviews.

In summary, when feedback is used to alter physicians' practice patterns, the programs are most likely to be successful if the data are individualized, if doctors are compared with their peers, and if the information is delivered personally by a physician in a position of clinical leadership. As is the case with the use of education to change practice patterns, feedback is most likely to be successful when it addresses a single clinical problem about which physicians have reached consensus regarding standards of practice. Feedback also seems more successful for outpatient than inpatient services. Even so, the cost of personalized face-to-face feedback may not generate savings that exceed its cost.

References

1. Mistry, F.D., and J.S. Davis. Teaching efficient and effective utilization of the clinical laboratory. *J. Med. Educ.* 1981; 56:356–58.

2. Boyd, J.C., D.E. Bruns, B.W. Renoe, J. Savory, and M.R. Witts. Medical education in laboratory testing: An approach incorporating the student's own laboratory results. *Am. J. Clin. Pathol.* 1983; 79:211–16.

3. Williamson, J.W., D.M. Barr, E. Fee, et al. *Teaching Quality Assurance and Cost Containment in Health Care: A Faculty Guide.* San Francisco: Jossey-Bass, 1982.

4. Williamson, J.W., J.I. Hudson, and M.M. Nevins. *Principles of Quality Assurance and Cost Containment in Health Care.* San Francisco: Jossey-Bass, 1982.

5. Weitberg, A.B. Laboratory testing in teaching hospitals: Impact on the cost of health care. *R.I. Med. J.* 1980; 63:441–42.

6. Smith, S.R. An evaluation of computerized exercise in teaching cost consciousness. *J. Med. Educ.* 1983; 58:146–48.

7. Fowkes, F.G.R., L.A. Williams, B.R.B. Cooke, R.C. Evans, S.H. Gehlbach, and C.J. Roberts. Implementation of guidelines for the use of skull radiographs in patients with head injuries. *Lancet.* 1984; 2:795–96.

8. Brook, R.H., K.N. Williams, and J.E. Rolph. Controlling the use and cost of medical services: The New Mexico Experimental Medical Care Review Organization—a four year case study. *Med. Care.* 1978; 16(suppl):1–76.

9. Brook, R.H., K.N. Williams, and J.E. Rolph. Use, costs, and quality of medical services: Impact of the New Mexico Peer Review System: A 1971–1975 study. *Ann. Intern. Med.* 1978; 89:256–63.

10. Brook, R.H., and K.N. Williams. Effect of medical care review on the use of injections: A study of the New Mexico Experimental Medical Care Review Organization. *Ann. Intern. Med.* 1976; 85:509–15.

11. Schroeder, S.A., L.P. Myers, S.J. McPhee, et al. The failure of physician education as a cost containment strategy: Report of a prospective controlled trial at a university hospital. *J.A.M.A.* 1984; 252:225–30.

12. Williams, S.V., and J.M. Eisenberg. Decreasing diagnostic test utilization. *J. Gen. Intern. Med.* 1986; 1:8–13.

13. Williams, S.V., J.M. Eisenberg, D.S. Kitz, et al. Teaching cost-effective diagnostic test use to medical students. *Med. Care.* 1984; 22:535–42.

14. Wong, E.T., M.M. McCarron, and S.T. Shaw, Jr. Ordering of laboratory tests in a teaching hospital: Can it be improved? *J.A.M.A.* 1983; 249:3076–80.

15. McDonald, C.J., S.L. Hui, D.M. Smith, et al. Reminders to physicians from an introspective computer medical record: A two-year randomized trial. *Ann. Intern. Med.* 1984; 100:130–38.

16. Davis, D., R.B. Haynes, L. Chambers, V.R. Neufield, A. McKibbon, and P. Tugwell. The impact of CME: A methodological review of the continuing medical education literature. *Eval. Health Prof.* 1984; 7:251–83.

17. Soumerai, S.B., and J. Avorn. Efficacy and cost-containment in hospital pharmacotherapy: State of the art and future directions. *Milbank Mem. Fund Q.* 1984; 62:447–74.

18. See reference 15 above.

19. Geertsma, R.H., R.C. Parker, Jr., and S.K. Whitbourne. How physicians view the process of change in their practice behavior. *J. Med. Educ.* 1982; 57:752–61.

20. Griner, P.F. Use of laboratory tests in a teaching hospital: Long-term trends—reductions in use and relative cost. *Ann. Intern. Med.* 1979; 90:243–48.

21. Grossman, R.M. A review of physician cost-containment strategies for laboratory testing. *Med. Care.* 1983; 21:783–802.

22. Everett, G.D., C.S. de Blois, P.F. Chang, and T.D. Holets. Effect of cost education, cost audits, and faculty chart review on the use of laboratory services. *Arch. Intern. Med.* 1983; 143:942–44.

23. Schroeder, S.A., K. Kenders, J.K. Cooper, and T.E. Piemme. Use of laboratory tests and pharmaceuticals: Variation among physicians and effect of cost audit on subsequent use. *J.A.M.A.* 1973; 225:969–73.

24. Cumming, K.M., K.B. Frisof, M.J. Long, and G. Krynkiewich. The effect of price information on physicians' test ordering behavior: Ordering of diagnostic tests. *Med. Care.* 1982; 20:293.

25. Long, M.J., K.M. Cummings, and K.B. Frisof. The role of perceived price in physicians' demand for diagnostic tests. *Med. Care.* 1983; 21:243–50.

26. Cohen, D.I., P. Jones, B. Littenberg, and D. Neuhauser. Does cost information availability reduce physician test usage? A randomized clinical trial with unexpected findings. *Med. Care.* 1982; 20:286–92.

27. Rhyne, R.L., and S.H. Gehlbach. Effects of an educational feedback strategy on physician utilization of thyroid function panels. *J. Fam. Pract.* 1979; 8:1003–7.

28. Freeman, R.A. Cost containment. *J. Med. Educ.* 1976; 51:157–58.

29. Lyle, C.B., Jr., R.F. Bianchi, J.H. Harris, and Z.L. Wood. Teaching cost containment to house officers at Charlotte Memorial Hospital. *J. Med. Educ.* 1979; 54:856–62.

30. See reference 24 above.

31. See reference 7 above.

32. See reference 17 above.

33. See reference 17 above.

34. Gryskiewicz, J.M., and D.E. Detmer. Waste not, want not: Use of blood in elective operations—improved utilization of blood by use of blood-ordering protocols and the type and screen. *Curr. Surg.* 1983; 40:371–77.

35. Williams, S.V., J.M. Eisenberg, D.S. Kitz, et al. Teaching cost-effective diagnostic test use to medical students. *Med. Care.* 1984; 22:535–42.

36. See reference 8 above.

37. See reference 4 above.

38. Eisenberg, J.M. Physician utilization: The state of research about physicians' practice patterns. *Med. Care.* 1985; 23:461–83.

39. Hale, F.A., K.C. Stone, D.J. Serbert, and E.C. Nelson. A clinical cost-consciousness learning packet for community-based clerkships. *Fam. Med.* 1984; 16:131–33.

40. Freymann, J.G. Teaching economic reality to medical students. *Bus. Health.* 1985; (April):14–18.

41. See reference 40 above.

42. See reference 15 above.

43. Wilson, G.A., C.J. McDonald, and G.P. McCabe, Jr. The effect of immediate access to a computerized medical record on physician test ordering: A controlled clinical trial in the emergency room. *Am. J. Public Health.* 1982; 72:698–702.

44. Johnson, M.W., W.E. Mitch, A.H. Heller, and R. Spector. The impact of an educational program on gentamicin use in a teaching hospital. *Am. J. Med.* 1982; 73:9–14.

45. See reference 40 above.

46. Cebul, R.D., and L.H. Beck. *Teaching Clinical Decision Making.* New York: Praeger Publishing. 1986.

47. Goodspeed, R., F. Davidoff, M. Testa, and J. Clive. "Little ticket" laboratory tests: Differential effect of probabilistic vs. cost-control curriculum on ordering rates [Abstract]. *Clin. Res.* 1985; 33:721A.

48. See reference 17 above.

49. Marton, K.I., V. Tul, and H.C. Sox. Modifying test-ordering behavior in the outpatient medical clinic: A controlled trial of two educational interventions. *Arch. Intern. Med.* 1985; 145:816–21.

50. Sanazaro, P.J. Determining physicians' performance: Continuing medical education and other interacting variables. *Eval. Health Prof.* 1983; 6:197–210.

51. Stross, J.K., and G.G. Bole. Evaluation of a continuing education program in rheumatoid arthritis. *Arthritis Rheum.* 1980; 23:846–49.

52. Stross, J.K., R.G. Hiss, C.M. Watts, W.K. Davis, and R. McDonald. Continuing education in pulmonary disease for primary-care physicians. *Am. Rev. Respir. Dis.* 1983; 127:739–46.

53. Thompson, R.S., H.L. Kirz, and R.A. Gold. Changes in physician behavior and cost savings associated with organizational recommendations on the use of "routine" chest x-rays and multichannel blood tests. *Prev. Med.* 1983; 12:385–96.

54. Check, W.A. How to affect antibiotic prescribing practices. *J.A.M.A.* 1980; 244:2594–95.

55. See reference 54 above.

56. See reference 19 above.

57. Winkler, J.D., K.N. Lohr, and R.H. Brook. Persuasive communication and medical technology assessment. *Arch. Intern. Med.* 1985; 145:314–17.

58. See reference 17 above.

59. Melmon, K.L., and T.F. Blaschke. The undereducated physician's therapeutic decisions. *N. Engl. J. Med.* 1983; 308:1473–74.

60. Avorn, J., and S.B. Soumerai. Improving drug-therapy decisions through educational outreach: A randomized controlled trial of academically based 'detailing.' *N. Engl. J. Med.* 1983; 308:1457–63.

61. Schaffner, W., W.A. Ray, C.F. Federspiel, and W.O. Miller. Improving antibiotic prescribing in office practice: A controlled trial of three educational methods. *J.A.M.A.* 1983; 250:1728–32.

62. See reference 61 above.

63. Ray, W.A., W. Schaffner, and C.F. Federspiel. Persistence of improvement in antibiotic prescribing in office practice. *J.A.M.A.* 1985; 253:1774–76.

64. Avorn, J., and S.B. Soumerai. A new approach to reducing suboptimal drug use. *J.A.M.A.* 1983; 250:1752–53.

65. Berner, E.S., L.R. Coulson, and B.P. Schmitt. A method to determine attitudes of faculty members toward use of laboratory tests. *J. Med. Educ.* 1985; 60:374–78.

66. Kassebaum, D.G. Teaching laboratory test use. *J. Med. Educ.* 1985; 60:420–21.

67. Altman, L.K. Prank punishes young surgeons. *New York Times.* 1984 September 4.

68. Stein, L.S. Education of residents [Letter]. *J.A.M.A.* 1981; 246:1299.

69. See reference 50 above.

70. See reference 8 above.

71. Hughes, R.A., P.M. Gertman, J.J. Anderson, et al. The Ancillary Services Review Program in Massachusetts: Experience of the 1982 pilot project. *J.A.M.A.* 1984; 252:1727–32.

72. See reference 12 above.

73. Eisenberg, J.M. An educational program to modify laboratory use by house staff. *J. Med. Educ.* 1977; 52:578–81.

74. Nelson, R.B. Teaching technologic restraint: An evaluation of a single session. *Eval. Health Prof.* 1978; 1:21–28.

75. See reference 27 above.

76. See reference 74 above.

77. See reference 73 above.

78. See reference 74 above.

79. Nanji, A.A. Medical grand rounds and laboratory use. *J.A.M.A.* 1983; 249:2890.

80. See reference 63 above.

81. Berbatis, C.G., M.J. Maher, R.J. Plumridge, J.U. Stoelwinder, and S.R. Zubrick. Impact of a drug bulletin on prescribing oral analgesis in a teaching hospital. *Am. J. Hosp. Pharm.* 1982; 38:98–100.

82. Everett, G.D., C.S. de Blois, and P.F. Chang. Impact of medical school

laboratory courses and physician attitude on test use by house staff. *J. Med. Educ.* 1983; 58:736–38.

83. Martin, A.R., M.A. Wolf, L.A. Thibodeau, V. Dzau, and E. Braunwald. A trial of two strategies to modify the test-ordering behavior of medical residents. *N. Engl. J. Med.* 1980; 303:1330–36.

84. See reference 13 above.

85. Restuccia, J.D. The effect of concurrent feedback in reducing inappropriate hospital utilization. *Med. Care.* 1982; 20:46–62.

86. Ende, J. Feedback in clinical medical education. *J.A.M.A.* 1983; 250:777–81.

87. See reference 20 above.

88. Fineberg, H.V., A.R. Funkhouser, and H. Marks. Variation in medical practice: A review of the literature. Presented at the Conference on Cost-Effective Medical Care: Implications of Variation in Medical Practice; Institute of Medicine, National Academy of Sciences, Washington, D.C.; February 1983.

89. Myers, L.P., and S.A. Schroeder. Physician use of services for the hospitalized patient: A review, with implications for cost containment. *Milbank Mem. Fund Q.* 1981; 59:481–507.

90. Eisenberg, J.M., and S.V. Williams. Cost containment and changing physicians' practice behavior: Can the fox learn to guard the chicken coop? *J.A.M.A.* 1981; 246:2195–2201.

91. Eisenberg, J.M. Modifying physicians' patterns of laboratory use. In Connelly, D.P., E.S. Benson, M.D. Burke, and D. Fenderson, eds. *Clinical Decisions and Laboratory Use.* Minneapolis: University of Minneapolis Press, 1982; 145–58.

92. See reference 88 above.

93. See reference 23 above.

94. See reference 14 above.

95. See reference 49 above.

96. Young, D.W. An aid to reducing unnecessary investigations. *Br. Med. J.* 1980; 281:1610–11.

97. See reference 11 above.

98. See reference 12 above.

99. Koepsell, T.D., A.L. Gurtel, P.H. Diehr, et al. The Seattle evaluation of computerized drug profiles: Effects on prescribing practices and resource use. *Am. J. Public Health.* 1983; 73:850–55.

100. See reference 17 above.

101. See reference 54 above.

102. Hillman, R.S., S. Helbig, S. Howes, J. Hayes, D.M. Meyer, and J.R. McArthur. The effect of an educational program on transfusion practices in a regional blood program. *Transfusion.* 1979; 19:153–57.

103. Rosser, W.W. Using the perception-reality gap to alter prescribing patterns. *J. Med. Educ.* 1983; 58:728–32.

104. Gehlbach, S.H., W.E. Wilkinson, W.E. Hammond, et al. Improving drug prescribing in a primary care practice. *Med. Care.* 1984; 22:193–201.

105. See reference 27 above.

106. See reference 19 above.

107. Anderson, O.W., and M.C. Shields. Quality measurement and control in physician decision making: State of the art. *Health Serv. Res.* 1982; 17:125–55.

108. See reference 83 above.

109. Cohen, D.I., B. Littenberg, C. Wetzel, and D. Neuhauser. Improving physician compliance with preventive medicine guidelines. *Med. Care.* 1982; 20:1040–45.

110. See reference 22 above.

111. Heath, D.A., R. Hoffenberg, J.M. Bishop, M.J. Kendall, and O.L. Wade. Medical audits. *J. R. Coll. Phys.* 1980; 14:200–201.

112. Marcy, W.L., S.T. Miller, and R. Vander Zwaag. Modification of admission diagnostic test ordering by residents. *J. Fam. Pract.* 1981; 12:141–42.

113. See reference 54 above.

114. Rhee, S.O., R.D. Luke, and M.B. Culverwell. Influence of client/colleague dependence on physician performance in patient care. *Med. Care.* 1980; 18:829–41.

115. McConnell, T.S., P.R. Berger, H.H. Dayton, B.E. Umland, and B.E. Skipper. Professional review of laboratory utilization. *Hum. Pathol.* 1982; 13:399–403.

116. Chokshi, A.B., H.S. Friedman, M. Malach, B.C. Vasavada, and S.J. Bleicher. Impact of peer review in reduction of permanent pacemaker implantations. *J.A.M.A.* 1981; 240:754–57.

117. Wennberg, J.E., L. Blowers, R. Parker, and A.M. Gittelsohn. Changes in tonsillectomy rates associated with feedback and review. *Pediatrics.* 1977; 59:821–26.

118. Winickoff, R.N., K.L. Coltin, M.M. Morgan, R.C. Buxbaum, and G.O. Barnett. Improving physician performance through peer comparison feedback. *Med. Care.* 1984; 22:527–34.

119. Forrest, J.B., W.P. Ritchie, M. Hudson, and J.F. Harlan. Cost containment through cost awareness: A strategy that failed. *Surgery.* 1981; 90:154–58.

120. Grivell, A.R., H.J. Forgie, C.J. Fraser, and M.N. Berry. Effect of feedback to clinical staff of information on clinical biochemistry requesting patterns. *Clin. Chem.* 1981; 27:1717–20.

121. See reference 12 above.

122. See reference 11 above.

123. See reference 49 above.

124. Applegate, W.B., M.D. Bennett, L. Chilton, B.J. Skipper, and R.E. White. Impact of a cost containment educational program on housestaff ambulatory clinic charges. *Med. Care.* 1983; 21:486–96.

125. Adler, N.E., and A. Milstein. Evaluating the impact of physician peer

review: Factors associated with successful PSROs. *Am. J. Public Health.* 1983; 73:1182–85.

126. See reference 85 above.

127. Lipp, C.S. Peer review experiment succeeds in Delaware. *Bus. Health.* 1984; 1(6):21–24.

128. See reference 50 above.

129. McPhee, S.J., S.A. Chapman, L.P. Myers, S.A. Schroeder, and J.K. Leong. Lessons for teaching cost containment. *J. Med. Educ.* 1984; 59:722–29.

130. See reference 11 above.

131. See reference 83 above.

132. Gertman, P.M., A.C. Monheit, J.J. Anderson, J.B. Eagle, and D.K. Levenson. Utilization review in the United States: Results from a 1976–1977 national survey of hospitals. *Med. Care.* 1979; 17(suppl):1–148.

133. Smits, H.L. The PSRO in perspective. *N. Engl. J. Med.* 1981; 305:253–59.

134. Roberts, C.J., F.G. Fowkes, W.P. Ennis, and M. Mitchell. Possible impact of audit on chest x-ray requests from surgical wards. *Lancet.* 1983; 2:446–48.

135. Sherman, H. Surveillance effects on community physician test ordering. *Med. Care.* 1984; 22:80–83.

136. Devitt, J.E., and M.R. Ironside. Can patient care audit change doctor performance? *J. Med. Educ.* 1975; 50:1122–23.

137. See reference 127 above.

7

Other Approaches to Changing Physicians' Practices

Among medical educators and health services researchers, education and feedback have been the most popular approaches to modifying physicians' use of medical services. Admittedly, it is appealing to think that doctors will change their practice patterns without resistance once they are taught how these services should be provided and once they are given information about how their own practices compare with reasonable standards.

One of the reasons that these two approaches of education and feedback have been adopted so often is that they fit the professional model of medical decision making so nicely. If only doctors knew more about the value of the services they have available to them, goes the argument, they would use those services more appropriately. Given better epidemiologic and economic data and a few guidelines about how their peers practice, the doctors practicing at variance with these standards would come around quickly. These strategies assume that physicians are well motivated. They assume that physicians' basic, even if unrecognized, desires to provide value for money in medical care can be activated by making them aware of information about cost-effective practice, by informing them about the difference between their own practices and an ideal or norm.

Although this professional model of physician decision making is an attractive one, the data do not always bear it out. Numerous studies of programs using education and feedback have shown doctors to be

resistant to change. Since one might well suspect that these negative
studies reflect only some of the failures to change doctors' utilization
patterns because of the frequent and regrettable reluctance to publish
negative studies, we must look for additional ways to influence physicians' practices. Even when education and feedback are effective in altering doctors' practices, it is not clear that they are efficient. These strategies
for change can be time consuming and labor intensive; they often require
more energy, imagination, and leadership than are available.

Given the multiplicity of influences on medical care utilization, it
should be expected that a single approach to change is not consistently
effective. In any effort to modify doctors' practices, those planning the
intervention must understand why the doctors have chosen the services
they are prescribing. The intervention should be chosen to fit the reasons
for the doctors' behavior. If the remedy does not suit the illness, or if it
is implemented less than optimally, the result is likely to be failure.

In addition to education and feedback, several other approaches have
been used, including participation by doctors in the change efforts, administrative rules, financial incentives, and penalties. As Wennberg points
out, these other means of changing practice styles do not follow the professional model of the knowledgeable clinician decision maker [1]. They
either involve doctors in hospital administrative decisions, establish rules
that restrict the independence of doctors' decisions, or appeal to doctors'
personal financial interests. Although these interventions have not been
evaluated critically as often as education and feedback, they are increasingly being adopted by hospitals, third-party payers, health maintenance
organizations, and employers who are worried about the increasing cost
of medical care.

Participation

A corollary to the importance of involvement by clinical leadership in
feedback programs is the role of participation by physicians in any effort
to change practice patterns. The principles of management theory predict
that active participation by physicians in planning and implementing
programs to change utilization will contribute to their success. In general,
when a change in the behavior of professionals is desired, the professionals should be involved in the decision-making process. The more
ambiguous the task is and the more decentralized the activities of the
professionals are, the more they want and expect to have a voice in
changes that affect them. In more general terms, the strategy for change
should be designed to match the style that the object of the strategy finds

most comfortable. The success of participation in changing the practices of professionals who work with uncertain, ambiguous problems has also been shown to hold true for scientists in research laboratories. The principles of contingency theory, as described in chapter 5, would predict these results: that the style of management should be contingent on the nature of the people, the task, and the organization.

However, in the past, hospital administrators have seldom involved physicians in operational decisions. Hospitals have often operated as institutions with two parallel social and management structures—those of administration and of physicians—playing their separate roles in a "power equilibrium" [2].

The separation of the hospital into two spheres of influences, administrative and clinical, has affected the way doctors view the institution. Physicians have often perceived the hospital simply as their workshop and, generally, a rent-free workshop. The principal role of the hospital, so far as most physicians could tell, was to facilitate their practices or to place constraints on them [3]. Few physicians were involved in cost-containment efforts [4]. For the individual clinician, dealing with these larger issues of cost containment and resource allocation sometimes seemed to be in conflict with the Hippocratic commitment to the individual patient [5]. Weighing the social good with the patient's benefit was something physicians were uncomfortable doing.

Despite the usual absence of practicing physicians in the planning of cost-containment activities, there have been impressive exceptions. Stoelwinder and Clayton described a reduction in patient stays, reduced waiting time for emergency services, and a lower rate of increase for admission costs when physicians and hospital administrators worked together [6]. Berger has reported on the efforts of other hospitals and associations to involve physicians in these decisions [7].

The organization of the cost-containment effort at the Johns Hopkins Hospital in Baltimore is another example of successful participation by medical staff in a program designed to change practice patterns. In the late 1970s, as part of an effort to reduce costs, the hospital's management was decentralized into a series of functional units, each directed by one of the academic clinical chiefs. Using information systems to provide data, this "meeting of the barons" effectively involved physicians in the change process and was said to decrease the previously steep increase in hospital expenditures [8–11].

Similar results have been achieved by health maintenance organizations (HMO) that have enabled physicians to participate in efforts to change practice patterns. When HMO physicians are involved in admin-

istrative roles related to cost containment, reduced use of diagnostic testing is found [12]. Doctors in these organizations who report greater
participation in the management of their practices also are more satisfied
with their work [13]. One HMO used group decision making to develop
a new policy on preventive measures, such as the use of screening tests,
and reported savings of over $150,000. There was a fivefold decrease in
"nonindicated" chest radiology (from 29.8 percent to 6 percent) and a
reduction in the use of multichannel chemistry tests for routine office
examinations from 36 percent to 15 percent [14].

The value of physician involvement in efforts to change their practices is one of the most important lessons of the literature about quality
assurance. Although how to involve doctors in quality assurance and
when their participation should be elicited are questions of some controversy, there is general agreement that participation is important for the
program's success. Whether this involvement means allowing doctors to
set the criteria for quality assessment, to review clinical records, or simply
to share the data, physicians need to feel vested in the program in order
to respond optimally [15].

In anticipating the need for more physician participation in cost-
control programs with the introduction of case-mix-based prospective
reimbursement (such as those using diagnosis related groups), Young
and Saltman have proposed that incorporating doctors into the management control system will be the key to cost-containment efforts [16, 17].
They point out the need for "goal congruence," or agreement on the target
of the change process, by physicians and administrators. The importance
of participation by physicians (or the "pantisocratic approach" to management) has also been emphasized for educational programs [18, 19].

Accordingly, the advent of prospective payment has induced hospital administrators to become more serious about involving physicians
in the management of the hospital, even if that means the hospital manager must relinquish a certain amount of control [20]. Some have called
for new ways of organizing the medical center, such as hospital-physician
joint ventures [21], to accomplish what Paul Ellwood [22] has described
as the "diplomatic miracle" of persuading doctors to control utilization.

One example of this sharing of control and involvement of physicians in hospital management is involvement of physicians on hospital
governing boards. A survey by the American Hospital Association in
1982 showed that 98 percent of responding hospitals had physicians on
the governing board up from 67 percent in 1973. In nearly every hospital,
the physician board members were also members of the hospital's medical
staff and served on the board with a vote [23].

Administrative Rules

An alternative to convincing physicians to change their practices is forcing the change through administrative fiat. When administrative rules make it impossible for physicians to practice in certain ways, it is no longer necessary to educate them to change their behavior or to give them feedback about their practices. Even so, administrative rules are most likely to be accepted if physicians understand the reasons for the changes and participate in their development.

Probably the most common example of administrative rules that restrict physicians' practices is the hospital formulary. When a hospital's pharmacy committee limits the drugs or brands of drugs that are available, whether for reasons of quality or cost containment, physicians' prescribing patterns are potentially altered. Even when the hospital pharmacy does stock a drug, a prescribing physician may need to obtain consultation to be allowed to prescribe it. This restriction is often instituted for new drugs, particularly antibiotics, to prevent biological resistance to the antibiotic by hospital organisms [24]. For example, when one hospital required that a specialist review orders for newer, more expensive, or more toxic antibiotics, it experienced a 60 percent to 90 percent reduction in utilization [25].

In addition to rules that restrict the use of drugs, simply changing the form that physicians use to order drugs may alter their prescribing patterns. In one hospital, a new order form obliged physicians to categorize antibiotic use as prophylactic, empirical, or therapeutic. When a drug was used for prophylaxis, the nurses were instructed to stop the drug therapy automatically after two days. When a drug was used for empirical therapy (treatment without knowledge of the organism responsible for the infection), the nurses were to stop therapy after three days. When the drug was used to treat a documented infection, therapy was stopped after seven days unless it was reordered. On the surgical service of this hospital, the use of antibiotics decreased dramatically with these administratively established rules and appropriate use increased [26].

Similar experiences have been reported with administrative rules designed to alter the use of diagnostic tests. Restrictions on laboratory test use by housestaff in medicine training programs at Duke, Stanford, and Rochester Universities contributed to a decrease in the use of tests [27–29]. However, when the medical board of a large, urban teaching hospital decided that standing orders were a cause of unnecessary diagnostic test use and eliminated these orders, no difference was seen in the total number of tests performed (although the use of chest radiographic examinations and electrocardiograms in the intensive care unit did decrease). Apparently, physicians simply wrote many more individual requests for tests that they would have otherwise obtained through standing orders [30]. This study illustrates the "balloon theory" of cost containment: if you squeeze it one place, it simply pops out at another.

Another system used to reduce diagnostic testing at many hospitals has been the institution of mechanisms of triage for those diagnostic services that seem to be overused, such as computed tomographic scans of the head or extensive analyses of clotting function. In these triage systems, physicians must receive approval for use of the test from a specialized physician on the hospital staff, such as a neurologist or neurosurgeon for head scans.

As in the case with prescription of drugs, another way to use administrative rules to alter laboratory test use is simply changing the request forms. Wong and colleagues showed that revising forms for requesting laboratory determinations of thyroid hormone levels led to a 38 percent decrease for triiodothyronine radioimmunoassay (measurement of a type of thyroid hormone) and a 61 percent decrease for measurement of thyrotropin levels (a hormone involved in thyroid control) [31]. This decrease was not observed in two control tests, one for which the order form was not changed and the other for which an educational program was instituted.

This strategy of changing the way that ancillary services are prescribed has been used for other services than diagnostic tests and drugs. One hospital, frustrated by the inappropriate ordering of blood for transfusions, established an automatic ordering system for blood. Instead of allowing doctors to decide whether to order cross-matched units or a "type and screen" (in which case blood is not matched nor is it held aside until it is needed), the blood bank used an algorithm to decide depending on the type of surgery planned. The proportion of cross-matched units fell dramatically [32].

Still another administrative rule to contain costs is to change the physician who is responsible for ordering tests. The success of the cost-containment program at Strong Memorial Hospital was associated with the replacement of junior residents by senior residents as supervisors of interns [33]. The literature on differences in diagnostic test use among physicians with different levels of experience, knowledge, and clinical maturity would predict reduced testing with this change in the assignment of residents. Interns who are supervised by more senior physicians would probably be advised to order fewer tests. In another study, when attending physicians were placed in charge of laboratory test ordering on teaching hospital wards, test ordering decreased 20 percent [34]. The reduction in tests ordered was most marked during the first four days of a patient's hospitalization, when screening tests of questionable use tend to be ordered.

Administrative rules designed to change practice patterns have also been introduced by third-party payers. For example, Blue Cross publicized its decision not to pay for on-admission tests unless the tests had been specifically prescribed for the patient by a physician. Previously, many hospitals had performed a battery of routine tests for all admitted patients, regardless of the patient's problem or whether the physician wanted the test.

Programs designed to give second opinions about surgery have also been instituted by those who would be responsible for paying for the surgery. Although the role of peer pressure and professional influence is certainly important in the effectiveness of second-opinion programs designed to decrease surgical utilization, the administrative requirement itself is responsible for part of the 15 percent to 25 percent reduction in rates of surgery [35]. The benefit-to-cost ratio of second-opinion surgery programs suggests that they save money despite their considerable expense. A mandatory second-opinion surgery program that had a 16 percent nonconfirmation rate reported a benefit-to-cost ratio of 2.63 [36]. A benefit-to-cost ratio between 3 and 4 was described for a Massachusetts second-opinion program that had a nonconfirmation rate of 14.5 percent [37].

Despite the apparent success of these administrative programs to alter practice patterns, use of this strategy may have risks. The restrictions are often so unpopular that they have to be discontinued. In addition to the possibility of an angry backlash by physicians if the administrative rules are capricious and not developed with the medical staff, the rules could also interfere with the quality of care and, in the long run, lead to increased costs [38, 39]. It is also possible that physicians will formally abide by the new regulations but circumvent them by prescribing other services that can substitute for the restricted ones. Even when the administrative rules appear to reduce utilization, they do not seem to affect underlying practice patterns. As is the case with the overweight person who loses weight on a crash diet, when administrative rules are relaxed, consumption often returns to its previous levels [40–42]. It is unclear whether administrative rules can ever be removed without losing the savings that were made by restricting doctors' decision making. To address these questions, adequately controlled research trials are needed to evaluate the impact of administrative rules that may seem at first to reduce unnecessary utilization [43].

Financial Incentives

The use of education, feedback, and physician participation to change the prescription of medical services suggests that doctors' practice patterns can be altered by programs that appeal to their desires to practice optimally, to serve as their patients' ideal agents, and to maintain position and stature among fellow professionals. The physician's financial self-interest does not play a role in these interventions, except to the extent that physicians want to win favor from patients and colleagues to increase income from future practice. Other programs to change physicians' practice patterns have appealed more directly to their economic desires and needs.

One way that programs have appealed to doctors' personal economic motivations is by offering financial incentives. Several plans have been tried, including the experimental program of Pennsylvania Blue Shield to pay physicians on a per-case basis, as described in chapter 2. This program had a small (3 percent) but statistically significant decrease in hospital costs. Because physicians were paid a lump sum for each patient with one of a variety of selected diagnoses, they no longer had incentives to prolong length of stay. This style of payment was similar to the way surgeons have been paid traditionally and the way hospitals are paid in the diagnosis related group prospective payment system [44]. Similar changes have been considered by the Health Care Financing Administration in which physicians would be prospectively paid a fixed amount per hospitalized patient. Although the Pennsylvania Blue Shield experiment suggests that hospital expenditures may be reduced slightly with prospective payment, little other evidence indicates that physicians will hospitalize their patients less. In fact, a prospective payment system has the potential disadvantage of offering physicians incentives to hospitalize patients for short stays and they could thereby reduce the threshold for admission. This would obviously result in more admissions, albeit with shorter lengths of stay, and hospital costs could paradoxically increase.

Part of the success of the decentralization of the Johns Hopkins Hospital and the concurrent involvement of clinical leadership may have been the financial incentives for the clinical departments to save money. Each department served as a cost center and had a voice in how their surpluses would be spent [45]. Similar projects incorporating physician involvement and the sharing of savings have been used in England under the leadership of Iden Wickings and the King's Fund.

On the other hand, financial incentives have generally not been successful in changing residents' utilization with the exception of Hunt's study, which was actually designed to increase productivity, not reduce costs [46]. The failure of programs that have used financial rewards to decrease laboratory testing by residents could have been due, in part, to differences between physicians in training and physicians in practice. Clearly physicians in different settings have different motivations, and it should be evident that few residents expect to obtain much income during their training. In addition, it should not be surprising, given residents' desire for approval by their supervising physicians, that the most successful programs to change housestaff practices have been those that have actively employed faculty physicians in face-to-face feedback about residents' use of tests, and that programs using financial incentives have not been successful [47, 48].

The incentive programs for residents may also have failed because the reward was not large enough. In the face of limited time, uncertainty, and the psychological weight of the many layers of supervision, it is not surprising that the chance to win a textbook or receive a small cash prize would have little effect. Perhaps token rewards are destined to evoke token responses.

Although HMOs sometimes offer incentives to physicians if the program has a surplus or holds down costs, most observers have questioned whether these financial incentives are the critical variable in the ability of HMO programs to reduce costs. The professional ethos and cost-conscious environment of the HMO may be a more powerful factor than the chance of financial rewards [49]. However, this weak influence of financial incentives in HMO programs could be due to the frequently remote relationship between the doctors' own practice, the HMO balance sheet, and doctors' bonuses.

The weakness of the evidence for an important effect of financial rewards on utilization behavior by physicians could be because the idea has never been given a reasonable chance. (Much the same argument was made in the previous chapter with reference to educational interventions.) In addition to being remote, the incentives are often too small to matter. Despite early reports about the cost-containment success of the SAFECO program, in which primary care physicians in an individual practice association served as gatekeepers to patients' use of available medical care services, long-term analysis suggests that the program did not work as well as was initially thought. It is likely that the incentives were not large enough to induce a typical individual practitioner to change utilization patterns [50, 51]. This discouraging evidence about the ability of the gatekeeper approach to save money has not really suggested that incentives do not work, but rather that relatively small rewards keyed to a small portion of a physician's practice will seldom change the style of that practice.

Much of the controversy about the gatekeeper plan has less to do with the lack of evidence that it saves money than with the fears that it could induce underutilization. Given the present information about the weak effect of this mandated form of case management, these fears seem unwarranted [52]. Whereas the possibility of underuse of necessary services should be monitored, the alarms currently being sounded are most likely politically motivated objections by those who oppose the plan either out of self-interest, concern for patients' freedom of choice, or ignorance.

Like the evaluation of gatekeeper systems, results of an experiment by Blue Shield of Massachusetts were also inconclusive. Blue Shield offered six obstetrician/gynecologists incentive payments of five dollars for each one-tenth of a day reduction in average length of stay that they achieved below a target, multiplied times the number of eligible patients for whom they provided care in normal deliveries, cesarean sections, and hysterectomies. An incentive was also offered to patients. Although the doctors decreased their average length of stay for all three procedures, none of the differences was statistically significant [53].

Notably, information is lacking about the ability of directed physician incentives to reduce medical care costs at a time when new forms of physician reimbursement are being considered. If a system such as prospective payment by diagnosis related group is instituted for physicians (which political soothsayers were doubting in early 1986), it may be that the emerging financial incentives for the hospital, joined with similar incentives for the physician, along with other programs such as feedback and participation, will be more effective than any one approach alone. This improvement would particularly be true if previous efforts had experienced only modest or equivocal success because the professional environment was not yet receptive to the need for reducing costs. Interventions using education and feedback may be more successful in the future as financial limitations become more severe and physicians are more aware of the need to reduce costs. For example, doctors practicing in a preferred provider organization, who are marketing their care as being less expensive, may be particularly interested in ways of cutting costs while maintaining (or even improving) quality. In fact, reductions in the number of hospital days used since the advent of prospective hospital payment and in HMO-dominated areas such as Minneapolis-St. Paul suggest that physicians will respond as the environment changes.

Penalties

Although the behavior modification literature suggests that incentives are generally more effective than penalties and that penalties may have the undesirable side effect of backlash (both passive and active), there has been somewhat more experience with penalties than with incentives in changing physician behavior.

Buck and White showed, in an early study of the effect of financial penalties on medical practice, that penalties resulted in decreased use of office injections [54]. An experiment in New York City also showed decreases in billings after the institution of a monitoring system that included the use of financial penalties [55].

The New Mexico Experimental Medical Care Review Organization suggested that penalties had little additional effect beyond that of education and feedback [56–58]. However, the substantial effects of the feedback program may have been due to the physicians' knowledge that the threat of financial penalties lay in the future for physicians who did not respond to the feedback [59]. In a similar vein, a program of financial penalties, along with feedback, was effective in decreasing total billings to Blue Shield of Pennsylvania by physicians. The decreased use of services by doctors who were exposed to the feedback program also may have been related to their knowledge of the potential use of penalties at a later stage in the program [60].

Financial penalties have also been tried in Canada. Like other programs of penalties, the Ontario Health Insurance Plan used a claims monitoring system to identify physicians likely to have overused services. The number of claims that were judged to be unnecessary fell from 7.95 percent of all cases to 5.6 percent. In 180 of the 519 cases brought to the attention of the medical review committee, physicians were ordered to refund money [61].

In this Canadian utilization review program, as well as in most others that have involved penalties, a committee of peers reviews the case to ensure that physicians are not penalized merely on the basis of statistical variation. Because of the important role of these professional leaders, the effectiveness of these programs may be due to the combined effect of financial penalty and peer pressure.

Because of the need to manipulate large data bases and to involve professionals in the audit process, claims review with chart audit is often an expensive way to reduce hospital costs. These programs seem to recover funds through penalties that are generally less than the expense of operating the program. Tuohy has suggested that, on the basis of excess payments recovered, the claims review system with the threat of financial penalty hardly justifies its costs [62]. However, she argues that the real intent of the procedure is preventive, to reduce utilization by physicians before its level triggers an audit. However, this spillover, or sentinel effect, has been difficult to document. If it does exist, then perhaps "the juice is worth the squeeze" for the claims monitoring programs, particularly if the system of penalties is combined with a program of education, feedback, and physician participation.

Ambiguous results were also obtained in the analysis of the Massachusetts Medicaid's reduction in physician fees on the use of surgery [63]. If subsequent studies show that targeted changes in physician fees can alter their practice styles, then this strategy might be used to reduce costs as well. Instead of the usual present schedule of physician fees, which encourages the use of procedures, a revised reimbursement scheme could be designed to encourage different levels and kinds of utilization.

Therefore, penalties do seem to be effective in changing physician practice patterns, whether as a threat or in actual application. In many instances of the successful application of penalties, the programs have been accompanied by other strategies to change physician practice. Given the complexity of physician behavior, it should not be surprising that a combined approach to change physicians' prescription of medical care is more often effective than programs that use one strategy alone.

The Underlying Principles: A Summary

The process of medical decision making is intriguingly complex. Although the emerging field of medical decision analysis is beginning to provide useful guidelines to aid clinical decision making, a variety of factors other than clinical logic influence physicians in their prescription of medical care. One set of influences includes those related to physicians' own self-interest. Desire for income, whether it be to maximize income or just to meet a target, is only one of the motives of self-fulfilling medical decision makers. Physicians are also strongly influenced by the style of practice to which they aspire (or that they want to maintain). Physicians' personal characteristics, such as specialty or age, and their practice settings also have marked effects on the prescription of medical services. Finally, the role of clinical leadership is a powerful influence on physicians' practice patterns.

In addition to physicians' self-interest, their commitment to their patients' well-being plays a major role in medical decision making. As their patients' agents, physicians will try to aid patients' economic well-being, especially in avoiding excessive out-of-pocket expenses. They will also consider clinical factors in deciding what they think is medically optimal care, but they do so in light of their perception of the patient's own desires for care and the patient's personal characteristics and convenience.

As the limitations on the social resources available for medical care become more widely recognized, physicians increasingly will face a third set of influences on their prescription of services: consideration of what is best for society as a whole. Whereas the physician's self-interest and the patient's benefit may sometimes conflict, the consideration of the scarcity of social resources for medical care presents the physician with the dilemma of weighing what seems to be best for the patient against what seems to be best for society.

The six major ways of altering physicians' practice patterns address these complex influences on medical decision making. Education, feedback, participation, administrative rules, incentives, and penalties may each address different factors that govern medical decision making. Any one by itself is less likely to be successful than an orchestrated combination. Although education may provide physicians with information to use in making better clinical decisions as their patients' agents (and to attract more patients), peer comparison feedback takes advantage of the important role of clinical leadership and the potency of the professional setting. Rewards and penalties use physicians' economic self-interest to shape their patterns of practice.

Fineberg and colleagues have offered an alternative framework for considering the influences on physicians' prescription of medical care [64]. They have summarized the underlying theories for physician decision making in three categories—cognitive, behavioral, and sociological—and have explained how the results of efforts to change behavior are consistent with this model. The cognitive theory treats the doctor as a processor of information. Physicians may have inaccurate information about the value of medical services, incomplete understanding of their patients' desires, or misperceptions of the actual clinical conditions of the patients. Even when physicians do have accurate information, they may handle it incorrectly or at least in different ways. If these inaccuracies and errors are a major reason for unnecessary use of services by physicians, then the appropriate intervention would be to educate physicians and give them feedback about differences between their behavior and optimal decision making.

The second theory that Fineberg and colleagues list is a behavioral one: physicians respond to the stimuli that they confront. These stimuli include the practice environment, patient demand, and financial incentives or penalties. According to this model, physicians may have accurate information and may be able to process it with facility, but they respond in understandable ways to the influences that face them in practice. To counter inappropriate behavior that is due to these influences, behavioral interventions should be instituted. These may involve altering the reimbursement incentives, instituting penalties in utilization review, or trying to change patients' expectations and desires.

The final theory proposed by Fineberg and colleagues is sociological. This model treats physicians as members of a social group. Physicians' practice patterns may be influenced by the physicians' own sociodemographic characteristics (for example, age) but are also influenced by their professional peer groups. This influence may occur as socialization during training or may take place later, as the physician is influenced by his peers in practice. Whereas some of these characteristics are fixed, others can be altered. To change physicians' practice patterns, it would be appropriate to use the strong influence of the norm of the professional peer group or attempt to change the group norm.

Undoubtedly, physicians today are more aware than ever before of the problem of medical care costs. The recent changes in Medicare reimbursement that introduced prospective payment by diagnosis related groups put pressure on hospitals to provide more efficient care, and hospital administrators are trying to enlist physicians in their new war on waste. At the same time, increasing competition from new forms of practice organization and payment for care, such as for-profit chains and preferred provider organizations, place pressure on physicians and hospitals to provide value for money in medical care. In this setting, where physicians are presumably more aware of the need to reconsider the efficiency of their practice styles, methods of changing their utilization of services may be more successful. The limited success of education and feedback in the past may have been due to the resistance of practitioners who were not ready to change. In a new era of medical practice in which cost is accepted as a factor to be considered, it may be that education, feedback, participation, administrative changes, incentives, and penalties will induce changes in utilization that were not achieved in the past.

Physicians' utilization of medical services is influenced by many diverse influences on clinical decision making. The black box of medical decision making does have windows through which we have come to understand some of the factors that shape this process. By understanding these influences, we can identify ways to alter them and change the decisions that govern the use of most medical care services.

References

1. Wennberg, J.E. On patient need, equity, supplier-induced demand and the need to assess the outcome of common medical practices. *Med. Care.* 1985; 23:512–20.

2. Young, D.W., and R.B. Saltman. Preventive medicine for hospital costs. *Harv. Bus. Rev.* 1983; 61:126–33.

3. Redisch, M. Physician involvement in hospital decision making. In Zubkoff, M., I.E. Raskin, R.S. Hanft, eds. *Hospital Cost Containment.* New York: Prodist, 1978; 217–43.

4. See reference 2 above.

5. Evans, R.W. Health care techology and the inevitabiltiy of resource allocation and rationing decisions: Part I. *J.A.M.A.* 1983; 249:2047–53.

6. Stoelwinder, J.U., and P.S. Clayton. Hospital organization development: Changing the focus from "better management" to "better patient care." *J. Appl. Behav. Sci.* 1978; 14:400–14.

7. Berger, J.D. Physician involvement in hospital cost control. *Hosp. Forum.* 1983; 26:17–21.

8. Johns, R.J., and B.I. Blum. The use of clinical information systems to control cost as well as to improve care. *Trans. Am. Clin. Climatol. Assoc.* 1979; 90:140–42.

9. Zuidema, G.D. The problem of cost containment in teaching hospitals: The Johns Hopkins experience. *Surgery.* 1980; 87:41–45.

10. Solomon, S. How one hospital broke its inflation fever. *Fortune.* 1979; 99:148–54.

11. Heyssel, R.M., J.R. Gaintner, I.W. Kues, A.A. Jones, and S.H. Lipstein. Decentralized management in a teaching hospital. *N. Engl. J. Med.* 1984; 310:1477–80.

12. Pineault, R. The effect of prepaid group practice on physicians' utilization behavior. *Med. Care.* 1976; 14:121–36.

13. Barr, J.K., and M.K. Steinberg. Professional participation in organizational decision making: Physicians in HMOs. *J. Community Health.* 1983; 8:160–73.

14. Thompson, R.A., H.L. Kirz, and R.A. Gold. Changes in physician behavior and cost savings associated with organizational recommendations on the use of "routine" chest x-rays and multichannel blood tests. *Prev. Med.* 1983; 12:385–96.

15. Sommers, L.S., R. Sholtz, R.M. Shepherd, and D.B. Starkweather. Physician involvement in quality assurance. *Med. Care.* 1984; 22:1115–38.

16. See reference 2 above.

17. Young, D.W., and R.B. Saltman. Medical practice, case mix, and cost containment: A new role for the attending physician. *J.A.M.A.* 1982; 247:801–5.

18. Williamson, J.W., D.M. Barr, E. Fee, et al. *Teaching Quality Assurance and Cost Containment in Health Care: A Faculty Guide.* San Francisco: Jossey-Bass, 1982.

19. Williamson, J.W., J.I. Hudson, and M.M. Nevins. *Principles of Quality Assurance and Cost Containment in Health Care.* San Francisco: Jossey-Bass, 1982.

20. Spivey, B.E. The relation between hospital management and medical staff under a prospective-payment system. *N. Engl. J. Med.* 1984; 310:984–86.

21. Shortell, S.M., T.M. Wickizer, and J.R.C. Wheeler. *Hospital-Physician Joint Ventures: Results and Lessons from a National Demonstration in Primary Care.* Ann Arbor, Mich.: Health Administration Press, 1984.

22. Ellwood, P.M. When MDs meet DRGs. *Hospitals.* 1983; 57(Dec. 16):62–66.

23. Noie, N.E., S.M. Shortell, and M.A. Morrisey. A survey of hospital medical staffs. *Hospitals.* 1983; 57(Dec. 1):80–83.

24. Check, W.A. How to affect antibiotic prescribing practices. *J.A.M.A.* 1980; 244:2594–95.

25. McGowan, J.E., and M. Finland. Usage of antibiotics in a general hospital: Effect of requiring justification. *J. Infect. Dis.* 1974; 130:253–59.

26. Durbin, W.A., Jr., B. Lapidas, and D.A. Goldmann. Improved antibiotic usage following introduction of a novel prescription system. *J.A.M.A.* 1981; 246:1796–1800.

27. Eisenberg, J.M., and S.V. Williams. Cost containment and changing physicians' practice behavior: Can the fox learn to guard the chicken coop? *J.A.M.A.* 1981; 246:2195–2201.

28. Griner, P.F. Use of laboratory tests in a teaching hospital: Long-term trends— reductions in use and relative cost. *Ann. Intern. Med.* 1979; 90:243–48.

29. Dixon, R.H., and J. Laszlo. Utilization of clinical chemistry services by medical house staff: An analysis. *Arch. Intern. Med.* 1974; 134:1064–67.

30. Sussman, E., P. Goodwin, and H. Rosen. Administrative change and diagnostic test use. *Med. Care.* 1984; 22:569–72.

31. Wong, E.T., M.M. McCarron, and S.T. Shaw, Jr. Ordering of laboratory tests in a teaching hospital: Can it be improved? *J.A.M.A.* 1983; 249:3076–80.

32. Gryskiewicz, J.M., and D.E. Detmer. Waste not, want not: Use of blood in elective operations: Improved utilization of blood by use of blood-ordering protocols and the type and screen. *Curr. Surg.* 1983; 40:371–77.

33. See reference 28 above.

34. Boice, J.L., and M. McGregor. Effect of residents' use of laboratory tests on hospital costs. *J. Med. Educ.* 1983; 58:61–64.

35. Vayda, E., and W.R. Mindell. Variations in operative rates: What do they mean? *Surg. Clin. North Am.* 1982; 62:627–39.

36. Ruchlin, H.S., M.L. Finkel, and E.G. McCarthy. The efficacy of second-opinion consultation programs: A cost-benefit perspective. *Med. Care.* 1982; 20:3–20.

37. Martin, S.G., M. Schwartz, B.J. Whalen, et al. Impact of a mandatory second-opinion program on Medicaid surgery rates. *Med. Care.* 1982; 20:21–45.

38. Lundberg, G.D. Laboratory request forms (menus) that guide and teach. *J.A.M.A.* 1983; 249:3075.

39. Brook, R.H., and K.N. Lohr. Second opinion programs: Beyond cost-benefit analyses. *Med. Care.* 1982; 20:1–2.

40. See reference 25 above.

41. McGowan, J.E., and M. Finland. Effects of monitoring the usage of antibiotics: An inter-hospital comparison. *South. Med. J.* 1976; 69:193–95.

42. Craig, W.A., S.J. Ulman, W.R. Shaw, V. Ramgopal, L.L. Eagan, and E.T. Leopold. Hospital use of antimicrobial drugs: Survey at 19 hospitals and results of antimicrobial control programs. *Ann. Intern. Med.* 1978; 89:793–95.

43. Rock, W.A., Jr., and J.E. Grogan. Demand versus need versus physician perogatives in the use of the WBC differential. *J.A.M.A.* 1983; 249:613–16.

44. Markel, G.A. Hospital utilization effects of case reimbursement for medical care. In Gabel, J.R., J. Taylor, N.T. Greenspan, and M.O. Blaxall, eds. *Physicians and Financial Incentives: Health Care Financing Conference Proceedings.* Washington, D.C.: Department of Health and Human Services, Health Care Financing Administration, 1978:95–99.

45. See reference 11 above.

46. Hunt, D.D. Effects of incentives on economic behavior and productivity of psychiatric residents. *J. Psychiatr. Educ.* 1980; 4:4–13.

47. Williams, S.V., J.M. Eisenberg, L. Poyss, and S.I. Rubin. Decreasing diagnostic test utilization [Abstract]. *Clin. Res.* 1981; 29:337A.

48. Martin, A.R., M.A. Wolf, L.A. Thibodeau, V. Dzau, and E. Braunwald. A trial of two strategies to modify the test-ordering behavior of medical residents. *N. Engl. J. Med.* 1980; 303:1330–36.

49. Luft, H.S. How do health-maintenance organizations achieve their "savings"? *N. Engl. J. Med.* 1978; 298:1336–43.

50. Moore, S. Cost containment through risk-sharing by primary care physicians. *N. Engl. J. Med.* 1979; 300:1359–62.

51. Moore, S.H., D.P. Martin, and W.C. Richardson. Does the primary-care gatekeeper control the costs of health care? Lessons from the SAFECO experience. *N. Engl. J. Med.* 1983; 309:1400–1404.

52. Eisenberg, J.M. The internist as gatekeeper. *Ann. Intern. Med.* 1985; 102:537–43.

53. Sims, P.D., D. Cabral, W. Daley, and L. Alfano. The incentive plan: An approach for modification of physician behavior. *Am. J. Public Health.* 1984; 74:150–52.

54. Buck, C.R., Jr., and K.L. White. Peer review: Impact of a system based on billing claims. *N. Engl. J. Med.* 1974; 291:877–83.

55. Paris, M., J. McNemara, and M. Schwartz. Monitoring ambulatory care: Impact of a surveillance program on clinical practice patterns in New York City. *Am. J. Public Health.* 1980; 70:783–88.

56. Brook, R.H., K.N. Williams, and J.E. Rolph. Controlling the use and cost of medical services: The New Mexico Experimental Medical Care Review Organization—a four year case study. *Med. Care.* 1978; 16(suppl):1–76.

57. Brook, R.H., K.N. Williams, and J.E. Rolph. Use, costs, and quality of medical services: Impact of the New Mexico Peer Review System—a 1971–1975 study. *Ann. Intern. Med.* 1978; 89:256–63.

58. Brook, R.H., and K.N. Williams. Effect of medical care review on the use of injections: A study of the New Mexico Experimental Medical Care Review Organization. *Ann. Intern. Med.* 1976; 85:509–15.

59. See reference 27 above.

60. Schwartz, J.S., S.V. Williams, J.M. Eisenberg, and D.S. Kitz. Effect of

utilization review on physician billings [Abstract]. *Med. Decis. Making.* 1981; 1:466.

61. Tuohy, C. Does a claims monitoring system influence high-volume medical practitioners? Attitudinal data from Ontario. *Inquiry.* 1982; 19:18–33.

62. See reference 61 above.

63. Schwartz, M., S.G. Martin, D.D. Cooper, G.M. Ljung, B.J. Whalen, and J. Blackburn. The effect of a thirty percent reduction in physician fees on Medicaid surgery rates in Massachusetts. *Am. J. Public Health.* 1981; 71:370–75.

64. Fineberg, H.V., A.R. Funkhouser, and H. Marks. Variation in medical practice: A review of the literature. Presented at the Conference on Cost-Effective Medical Care: Implications of Variation in Medical Practice, Institute of Medicine, National Academy of Sciences, Washington, D.C., February 1983.

Part III

Directions for Research
on Physician Utilization

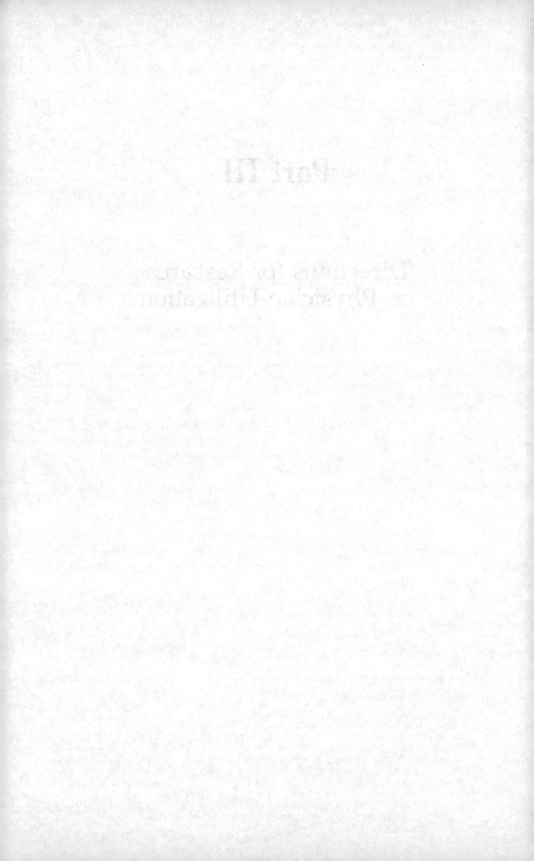

Efforts to open the black box of physician decision making have revealed a sometimes baffling array of influences. The physician cannot be envisioned simply as a creature of economic desires any more than as a self-sacrificing martyr for health or as one who makes impeccably logical decisions based on inarguable fact. The physician's desire to maximize personal utility may conflict with the interests of the patient, and both goals may conflict with the most efficient allocation of resources for social good. While a substantial amount of research has clarified the motivations for physicians' decisions to use medical services and has identified ways of changing their practice patterns, this work has been like most research—it raises more questions than it answers. The methodology of this research has become more refined, but health services researchers continue to develop new ways of better understanding doctors and their practices.*

---

*The following two chapters are adapted from the article from which this book developed (Eisenberg, J.M. Physician utilization: The state of research about physicians' practice patterns. *Med. Care.* 1985; 23:461–83). Portions of the article are reproduced with permission of the publisher of *Medical Care*.

8

Research and Physician Utilization

The principal approaches to research on physician utilization have included:

1. econometric models from aggregated data bases
2. small-area variation studies
3. national utilization surveys
4. analysis of claims data
5. use of clinical and management information systems
6. primary data collection at the level of the encounter

This chapter will discuss these approaches to investigation of physicians' practices, emphasize the methodologic issues they raise, and outline advances that are needed in this field of health care research.

Those who first studied physicians' practice patterns were often economists, and some of the earliest efforts to understand the interaction of the multiple influences on medical care utilization used complex mathematical models and intricate econometric methods [1].

Most of the econometric models have depended on large banks of aggregate data, particularly those available from Medicare and Medicaid and from a few national surveys. Figures on the utilization of certain services such as surgery have been available for analysis, but most data have been limited to information about total health care expenditures and its major components. Information on providers has often been limited to data about the number and types of physicians in certain locales and the number of hospital beds and their occupancy. With aggregate data like these, it has been possible to develop valuable models of how system-wide influences, such as alterations in reimbursement rates or changes in the supply of physicians, affect overall utilization, but it has been impossible to comment, except inferentially, on the doctor-patient interaction and on medical decision making.

Some progress was made in moving from this kind of macroanalysis of the factors that influence physicians' utilization to microanalysis when investigators began to study variations among small areas as a way of understanding medical care utilization. Data bases that characterize medical care services and resources in small areas, such as the Area Resource File of the Bureau of Health Professions and hospital-specific utilization data bases (for example, the Professional Activities Survey of the Commission on Professional and Hospital Activities), have been valuable in documenting small-area variation and in demonstrating that differences in utilization cannot entirely be explained by demographic or clinical differences of the populations. However, the data in these early studies of small-area variation were still aggregated and may have masked important differences among the smaller subunits: hospitals, doctors, and individual encounters. In addition, methodological problems such as defining a hospital's service area and taking into account the crossing of area borders by patients have hampered the application of small-area studies except in a few predominantly rural areas.

These early small-area analyses of utilization clearly documented the existence of variation among small areas, and recent work has begun to show differences among hospitals and even among individual physicians [2–4]. Attention is also now being directed at differences in clinical outcomes, such as surgical mortality, that are related to these differences in utilization.

Challenges for Research on Methodological Issues

While it is certainly important to study these differences in outcome and to determine whether they may be caused by differences in utilization, research is also needed to assess causation at a more fundamental level: what causes variation in utilization itself. If health care researchers can unravel the causes of this variation, they may be able to gain valuable insights into the underpinnings of medical decision making and ways to influence it. Several research areas which are most in need of methodological development are enumerated below:

1. evaluation and development of information sources (for example, claims data)
2. case mix and severity of illness measures
3. longitudinal data
4. need for prospective studies
5. ability to generalize
6. clarity of definitions
7. understanding the medical decision-making process
8. statistical properties of utilization data

Sources of Data

The National Center for Health Services Research, the National Center for Health Statistics, and others have made efforts to reveal the characteristics of medical care utilization at the level of the individual doctor and patient as a way of explaining differences in utilization. Several national surveys have collected information about the use of medical care services and their costs. For example, the National Ambulatory Medical Care Survey has made it possible to characterize and understand differences among physicians' utilization patterns at the level of the individual encounter. These encounter-specific data have enabled investigators to study differences in utilization and practice style, such as those among doctors of different specialties or different settings [5–7]. When diagnostic information has been included, the encounter-specific data bases have facilitated important efforts to control for case mix.

Another way to view the factors that influence decision making at the level of the individual case has been to analyze claims forms. Claims have been useful in assessing variation among small areas, hospitals, and physicians in hospital-based services for which claims are submitted. However, most hospital claims only record major procedures and many of the clinical components of care are aggregated into a total charge, such as that for all laboratory tests or all radiologic procedures. Sometimes more detailed information about utilization can be found in ambulatory claims. Because doctors must submit bills for ambulatory services on the basis of individual encounters and usually for specific ancillary services, these claims offer data more detailed than do areawide statistics or even hospital billings.

As information systems become more widely used by hospitals and other large practice organizations for both clinical and management information, it will be important to assess whether these local data bases offer opportunities beyond the scope of information from claims for understanding factors that affect physicians' practices. The computerization of billing services will be accompanied by the increased use of computers by hospitals to manage their internal operations, such as their ancillary service programs, and to provide clinical information to physicians. This information may also provide insights into physician decision making. A number of health maintenance organizations also have developed clinical and management data bases that offer opportunities for evaluation of the factors that influence physician utilization.

These new information systems, whether developed to record billings or to serve clinical or management purposes, provide access to encounter-specific utilization with which the physician's and the patient's characteristics, as well as other aspects of the encounter such as organizational and clinical factors, can be considered. The mass of data that is becoming available raises serious questions about whether the confidentiality of the doctor-patient relationship can be preserved, as well as whether the limitations of the data will be appreciated by those using them to probe the practice of medicine. Even encounter-specific data bases may be insufficient to understand the more subtle influences on medical decision making, be they cognitive, behavioral, or sociological [8]. In the end, primary data collection at the level of the doctor-patient interaction may be necessary to understand how the various influences on medical decision making explain variation in utilization.

Even with the promise of linkage of Medicare Part A and Part B files, a fuller understanding of the factors that influence the utilization of medical services will require information about services that are not available on current claims or in the current national reporting systems (for example, diagnostic tests and individual drugs for inpatients). Because of their increasing payments for medical care, businesses are now beginning to collect data on the utilization of medical services by employees, and this source of data may provide additional opportunities to study utilization in the detailed manner that is necessary.

However, as changes in arrangements to fix levels of payment for medical care, such as prospective payment of physicians and prepaid capitation plans, give providers incentives to improve their information systems for the purposes of internal management, these changes also will eliminate the necessity of billing for individual services. Therefore, at the same time that data on diagnoses and major procedures improve, a paradoxical decrease in available data about utilization could result, particularly about the use of "little-ticket" ancillary services such as diagnostic tests and drug prescriptions.

In addition to studying utilization data to understand differences among physicians and hospitals in their prescription and provision of medical care, researchers can use such information as feedback to change physicians' practices. This feedback can be delivered as periodic reports or with the use of computer terminals at which physicians order services (such as diagnostic tests or drugs) and can even be provided simultaneously with the request [9].

Despite the exciting potential for these sources of utilization information, such as claims data, in studying physician utilization patterns, much work remains to be done in assessing the validity and completeness of these data, as well as in using them to probe medical decision making. An inevitable tension exists between the need to carry out the critical methodological research that will provide the underpinnings of utilization studies and the enticing attraction of using the available data for substantive evaluations of what they mean. When John Naisbitt wrote in his best seller, *Megatrends*, "We are drowning in information but starved for knowledge," he was expressing concern about uncontrolled and unorganized data that could, if they were the manager's servant instead of master, provide valuable insights into how systems operate and how they can be improved [10]. The same concern about how information is used, and the opportunity to use it that is often lost, led T.S. Eliot to write, "Where is the wisdom we have lost in knowledge? Where is the knowledge we have lost in information?" [11].

Before the emerging volumes of data about utilization can be considered valuable, much will need to be done in evaluating the credibility of the information they contain and in developing ways of comprehending the messages that they may offer about how medical care is practiced. The main problem with claims forms is that, for all their detail, they may not be accurate, particularly with regard to diagnostic information. This problem is one of the most important of the methodological challenges facing researchers who study the factors that influence medical care utilization. For example, the discharge diagnoses that were listed in 1981 Medicare claims data for 32 community hospitals in the Minneapolis–St. Paul area generated diagnosis related groups (DRG) that agreed in only 53 percent of cases with the groups based on chart review [12]. The hospital-specific agreement rate ranged from 36 percent to 71 percent. The Institute of Medicine of the National Academy of Science has reported similar discrepancies in the coding of Medicare claims [13]. It found the reliability of diagnoses to be about 60 percent and the reliability of specific categories of procedures to range from 32 percent to 98 percent.

Claims forms for hospital services seem to be more complete in Canada than in the United States, but they still suffer inaccuracies. Roos and Roos have evaluated the data of the Manitoba Health Services Commission and concluded that the most accurate information is face sheet data and discharge status (alive or dead) [14]. Information about procedures that are performed in the hospital are less accurate, and diagnostic information presents the largest problem.

Bunker and colleagues have described some of the other methodological issues raised by the inaccuracies of claims forms, both those submitted by hospitals and those submitted by physicians (for example, occasional double insurance coverage of the patient, coding errors, and difficulty in coding new services) but have concluded that these forms can still be valuable in utilization research when used carefully [15].

Other problems with using claims data to investigate the utilization of medical care are the differences in coding procedures that are used by different fiscal intermediaries and the frequent coding of doctors in group practices together rather than individually. With more payers using DRG-based prospective payment, it is possible that more standard reporting is on the horizon and that providers will have reason to be more conscientious about their reporting accuracy. This is one of the charges from Congress to the new peer review organizations (PROs) and may facilitate comparisons across payment systems.

As third-party payers increasingly computerize their claims information, they offer more promise for studies of physician behavior. Claims data could be used to create profiles of physicians who practice similarly in order to characterize them. Do physicians who prescribe large or small numbers of certain services or physicians who use certain new, unusual, or outdated services have characteristics in common? Can groups of doctors who practice alike be clustered to define networks of physicians and to study the influences of team decision making, peer pressure, and clinical leadership in shaping practice patterns?

Claims data could also be used to characterize patients' clinical characteristics over time. For example, Roos has shown how claims in Manitoba, Canada, could define the prehysterectomy histories of women as well as to monitor these women for complications of the surgery [16].

Case Mix and Severity of Illness Measures

In addition to the need to continue investigating the potential usefulness and validity of large data bases, especially those based on claims, the methods now available to describe case mix and the severity of illnesses must be assessed and improved. Diagnosis related groups may make disease coding practical for reimbursement purposes by creating groups that are reasonably homogeneous according to length of stay, but the ability of these groups, or any case-mix system, to provide information about the severity of disease and the need for different levels of care will be critical in assessing physicians' utilization. The clinical homogeneity of these case-mix measures remains to be shown, even if the data are accurate. The study that showed only half of the DRG assignments in Minneapolis to be accurate showed that with more complete and accurate data, hospital case mix is on average about 4 percent more complex than the Health Care Financing Administration perceives it to be [17]. In some hospitals, the case mix was understated by as much as 15 percent.

Without a measure of the severity of illness, research that attempts to explain differences in physicians' utilization patterns will be confounded by the different types of clinical problems physicians confront. Recent progress has been substantial in this area, with important contributions by Horn, Young, and Gonnella, among others [18], but much work remains in developing measures of severity of illness that will facilitate better understanding of factors that influence medical decision making. Particularly important are systems that do not require costly collection of additional data from medical records, are related to the problems that patients present to the doctor (rather than the final diagnosis, which is probably less important in determining utilization than the presenting complaints), and are reproducibly collected from different settings.

Longitudinal Data

Several other areas of research in utilization merit methodological attention, in addition to those studying measures of case mix and severity of illness. For example, the existing literature on factors that influence physician utilization suffers from being a collection of snapshots at single points in time. Because almost all studies have been cross-sectional analyses, it has not been possible to observe the effects of long-term changes in the practice environment or to demonstrate the effect of physicians' personal maturation or change.

Cross-sectional variations among physicians' practices could be due to differing degrees of adoption of new practice patterns; perhaps ultimately almost all physicians will adopt the new style. For example, differences in average length of stay between hospitals on the East Coast and West Coast may simply signify that western physicians have adopted shorter lengths of stay more quickly that eastern physicians have, not that eastern physicians intrinsically use the hospital more. Perhaps the greater use of diagnostic tests in teaching hospitals is simply a harbinger of a changing practice style that all doctors will soon adopt, rather than evidence that teaching hospitals are inherently more expensive or less efficient.

This potential blindspot of cross-sectional studies, their inability to discriminate between differences that are intrinsic and those that are due to different stages of the same evolutionary process, has long been recognized by economists who study developing nations. These researchers have considered the possibility that all countries pass through the same developmental process and that comparative differences can be interpreted synchronically or diachronically, that is, in terms of differences between countries at one point in time or between the situations of a single country at successive times [19]. In biology, this paradigm has been described as ontogeny replicating phylogeny (the embryologic development of an individual mimics the evolutionary development of the species). Therefore, it will be necessary to observe changes in practice over time to understand decision making by physicians. Longitudinal studies will provide a more dynamic view of influences on physicians' use of medical care.

Need for Prospective Studies

It may be unrealistic to expect large data bases to provide information about doctors, patients, and their encounters if they do not serve the primary purpose of those who assembled the data bases. Because third-party payers are unlikely to be interested in identifying data such as the doctor's leadership role in the local hospital, many of the factors that are critical in influencing utilization levels will not be measured unless studies with that purpose are planned and performed. The risk of hypothesis hunting that exists when reams of data are forced into regression equations is less ominous when investigators decide on their research questions in advance of collecting data. Answers to complex questions such as the effect of financial incentives on physician behavior can be answered best by projects that control for as many other variables as possible and carefully collect the needed information. Even relatively simple questions, such as the influence of patients' demographic characteristics on physicians' decisions, require control for covariation (correlation between multiple factors that can obscure some causal relationships as well as suggest causality incorrectly in other relationships) that may be unattainable from ready-made data bases. The Rand Health Insurance Experiment, which was designed primarily to study the effect of different types of coverage on patient behavior, has demonstrated the value of prospective studies with carefully constructed data sets in understanding medical practice [20]. It has provided valuable insights into physician behavior as well as consumer behavior, but it has also served as an example of how expensive these studies can be.

Ability to Generalize

In the absence of prospective trials and in the face of the limited scope of data that can be analyzed retrospectively, most investigators have chosen the population of physicians that they will study on the basis of their ability to get information on practice patterns rather than their ability to generalize from the results that the data generate. For example, the emphasis of the available research on practice patterns of residents and their malleability to change far exceeds the relative importance of residents in the provision of medical care. Even if the habits that residents learn in training do foreshadow the way they will practice in the future, few investigators would suggest that residents are motivated by the same factors that influence community physicians [21].

Another popular object for study by the health services researcher has been the HMO. Even though HMO practitioners are mature clinicians (as opposed to housestaff), the very nature of the practice and their selection of an HMO career limit the degree to which conclusions about practice patterns in an HMO can be generalized to the rest of American medical practice. Because the financial, social, and clinical influences on utilization will differ in different settings, it is important that the practices of community physicians receive the kind of scrutiny that residents and HMO doctors have undergone.

Another methodological issue related to the generalizability of findings is whether reasonable surrogates can be found for actual practice behavior. Frequently, patient management problems or other simulated clinical situations are used to determine how physicians would respond with a real patient. One study showed that the agreement between these simulated cases and real data was significant but not overwhelming [22]. The problem remains, therefore, whether less costly ways can be found to measure physicians' practices than auditing their behavior in actual clinical situations.

Clarity of Definitions

As data are collected about decision making and about medical services in community practice, the definitions that are used must be explicit. For example, many studies have ignored the fundamental differences in training and style between general practitioners and family physicians and have considered them together in studies of interspecialty differences in utilization. Rossiter and Wilensky have provided an example of how careful definitions of patient-initiated and physician-initiated outpatient visits can help to separate the factors that influence physicians' decisions about utilization from factors that influence patients' decisions [23].

Nonphysician Clinicians

Another blindspot of the available literature is the definition of a "clinician." Few have studied the practice behavior of nonphysician clinicians. Bailit and colleagues' analysis of dental utilization has implied that factors influencing utilization by physicians are also important in dental practice [24]. Although a number of studies have concluded that nurse practitioners provide care of high quality, few have assessed decision making by nurse practitioners about the use of medical services. Studies of utilization by these nonphysicians offer an opportunity to understand clinical decision making in the perspective of interprofessional differences in knowledge, reimbursement, values, and style.

Understanding the Decision-Making Process

The capacity of health care researchers to understand the factors that influence utilization has also been limited by an incomplete understanding of the process of medical decision making. Much of the research in the field has been prescriptive, providing models for optimal practice behavior. Although these studies have been valuable in describing how medicine should be practiced, they have contributed less to an understanding of how medicine is practiced. Important lessons can be learned from descriptive research on decision making.

Elstein and colleagues have described the need to develop methods to probe the cognitive processes of the physician [25]. They have pointed out the need to assess the amount of distortion that occurs in decision making when it is observed by methods such as simulated cases, which can obviously be controlled to a degree that studies based on chart audits or large data bases cannot. In addition, little is known about how physicians deal with probabilities and how they weigh the risks and benefits of medical care as they make their clinical decisions. Even less is known about how sociocultural factors such as the patient's sex, age, or race influence physicians' decisions about utilization [26].

Statistical Considerations

Once reliable and valid data about physician utilization are available, interesting questions will remain regarding the statistical properties of these data. Bailit and Clive have shown that the different potential shapes of the utilization curve present different statistical challenges [27]. They describe several possibilities, including a Gaussian normal distribution, a short-tailed distribution, a long-tailed distribution, and a polymodal distribution. These different distributions of utilization data will have important implications on investigators' decisions about sampling, the types of services to study, and the establishment of norms. Fineberg and associates have suggested transforming the raw data to obtain a Gaussian distribution and then calculating a relatively stable measure of variation such as the coefficient of variation [28].

In addition to statistical considerations regarding the shape of the distribution of utilization rates, other statistical challenges stand to be addressed. One generally well-appreciated possibility is that of regression to the mean, by which outliers are likely to be closer to the mean on a second measure simply by chance. Diehr has commented on several other possibilities, including the problem that can occur when one patient receives the procedure of interest more than once, which violates the usual statistical assumption that rates are proportions [29]. She also points out that the denominator may be misleading if all people in a population are not candidates for a service (for example, women who have had hysterectomies are not candidates for another). Of most importance, Diehr also shows that chance alone can explain much of the observed variation in medical practice. For example, the ratio of the largest rate to the smallest would be 10.9 if 20 small areas of 1,000 people each were compared, given an underlying mean rate of 5/1,000 in all of the areas. Methods to standardize rates have been developed to provide better estimates for groups of rates, such as the "indirectly standardized ratio" [30] and the "systematic component of variation" [31].

Connor and Gillings have addressed another statistical issue in utilization studies: the problem of "ecological inference" [32]. This error in logic may occur when regression methods are used to analyze macrolevel data on length of stay from third-party payers (aggregated information) to draw microlevel conclusions about effects occurring among particular variables that influence length of stay at the level of the individual hospital.

Still another statistical problem with research on physician utilization is selecting the proper unit of analysis. Should change be measured in the total number of services, total cost of those services, average use by doctor, average use by patient, or some other measure of utilization? The answer depends on the goal of the study. Because we are most concerned with changes in physician decision making, the individual physician should be the focus of the measure [33]. Unfortunately, the physician is often not the focus. In one review of 28 studies on provider behavior that had been published in prestigious journals, 20 contained this "unit of analysis error" [34]. The major hypothesis was a statement about the behavior or professional performance of various types of health care providers. Either the experimental intervention was directed at the practitioner or the practitioner was a major source of variability in the outcome variable. However, the statistical test in 20 of these 28 studies used patient-related encounters or events as the unit of analysis. By artificially increasing the sample size, this flaw increases the likelihood of inferring that a difference between experimental and control populations of physicians exists when no true difference exists.

If teams of physicians or hospitals are actually the object of the intervention (which is especially important to consider when there is substantial shared decision making or influence of physicians by their peers), then even the individual physician may be an inappropriate statistical unit. In these cases, the team or the hospital may be the best unit of analysis [35].

Even with improved statistical methods, researchers are trying to hit a moving target. The underlying forces that drive medical decision making may not change, but the environment in which they take place will be changing dramatically. New payment systems will be introduced. Increased competition among physicians will place new pressure on them because of both the greater numbers of practitioners and evolving professional acceptance of overt competition (such as advertising). New organizational schemes will influence the sociological milieu of practice and the greater proportion of women in practice will change physicians' outlook on their careers. These changes will certainly influence the use of services and may give investigators the opportunity to study their effects as a way to gain insight into the factors influencing medical decision making.

Challenges for Research on Changing Utilization

The response of physicians to efforts to alter their practice patterns also presents an interesting challenge to health services researchers. Six of the more perplexing problems for investigators are:

1. shift in practice patterns versus normalization of outliers
2. measures of medical necessity and appropriateness
3. relative effectiveness of different approaches to alter practice
4. decay of change and return to old patterns; the need for long-term evaluation
5. cost-benefit ratio of programs to change utilization
6. effect on clinical and health status outcomes.

Who or What Has Changed?

After a program to alter practice patterns has been implemented, the researcher must decide whether the change observed is for a large number of physicians so that the standard of practice has shifted or if the change is limited to physicians whose practices made them outliers (so the distribution becomes narrower and taller but the modal practice style remains the same). The latter change, in which outliers conform to the group norm, would be expected in programs that use the influence of a group to induce change. However, reduction in rates of overutilization or underutilization could simply be due to the statistical artifact of regression to the mean. In assessing which doctors have changed in response to the intervention, it is also important to determine whether intervention effects have spilled over to doctors who did not receive the intervention (perhaps due to contamination) or to services that were not targeted (suggesting that doctors' overall practice, as well as their use of the service in question, may have changed). Furthermore, if only certain physicians change or if the use of only certain services changes, information about why overutilization might have existed and which interventions work best may be hidden in these results.

Medical Necessity and Appropriateness

When efforts to change physician behavior are analyzed, most investigators simply report changes in utilization rates rather than specifying whether changes occurred in underutilization or overutilization. Although some have assumed that high utilization implies unnecessary utilization, the evidence for this assumption is weak [36]. Similarly, the proportion of test results that are normal does not predict well the probability of inappropriate utilization [37]. Expert judgement has been used to assess the appropriateness of services, but additional research is necessary to evaluate the effectiveness and efficiency of medical care in order to make these judgements. Because the ultimate standard for the effectiveness of medical services should be their contribution to the well-being of the patients, clinical outcomes as well as economic outcomes are important for studies of programs designed to change physician behavior [38, 39].

Because of the importance of these clinical factors in understanding the potential consequences of physicians' practice patterns, the fields of health services research and clinical epidemiology both have much to offer. In addition to contributing to an understanding of the effect of variation in practice patterns, these fields may help to reduce the uncertainty among physicians that is responsible for some variation. Much remains to be learned about the natural history of disease, its response to therapy, and the potentially adverse effects of medical services. Few diagnostic tests have been subjected to intensive analysis of their effectiveness in diagnosing disease, not to mention their contribution to improved health. Advances in health economics are clarifying the true costs of medical care and their economic benefits. Research in ethics and medical decision making is enabling patients' preferences and values to be described and considered more fully and to help physicians deal more comfortably with the uncertainty that will remain in medical decision making.

Comparison of Approaches

Much has been learned about physician behavior from the successes and failures of efforts to change it. The potent effect of personal individualized feedback from a clinical leader is one clear lesson from the literature on physician change. The importance of participation and active involvement by respected clinicians in educational programs has also been demonstrated clearly. Nevertheless, the relative contributions of different ways to change physician behavior remain uncertain and the differences in the abilities of different interventions to influence different types of physicians have not been defined. No longer is it sufficient to measure the impact of one type of intervention on one type of doctor; comparative analyses are needed.

Long-Term Evaluation

In addition to the need for comparative analyses, long-term evaluations of methods to change practice patterns should be done. Few longitudinal data have been collected and the ability of change in practice patterns to persist rather than decay has only recently been appreciated in the literature. It is likely that reinforcement of changes in practice patterns will be needed, whether through continued education, repeated feedback, or ongoing financial incentives.

Cost-Benefit Ratio

Schroeder and colleagues have recently emphasized the importance of measuring whether savings from programs that change physicians' utilization of services justify their expense [40]. Although personal individualized feedback about performance from a clinical leader is effective, it is also expensive and the benefits may not substantially outweigh the costs.

Effect on Health Outcomes

Whether or not the economic benefits of efforts to change physicians' practices suggest that "the juice is worth the squeeze," the effect of these programs on health outcomes of patients deserves attention. In assessing whether changes in practice patterns are clinically beneficial, it is doubtful that gross outcomes such as mortality rates will be sensitive enough to show a substantial effect. Data bases have seldom been available to assess the possibility of changes in more subtle outcomes such as adverse effects of drugs, disability, or surgical complication rates. Without prospective collection of information at the level of the individual doctor-patient encounter, it will be difficult to identify outcomes such as health status from the patient's perspective. These outcomes are difficult enough to measure with observations and interviews of patients. Further work will be needed to develop instruments that can easily determine changes in the health status of patients that result from programs designed to alter physicians' practice patterns [41]. Even without these data, we should be able to use the clinical literature to select those practice patterns most likely to affect health outcomes (for example, cancer screening and appropriate drug prescribing) and to assess physicians' behavior in these areas.

Other Methodologic Issues

Continued attention to the methodology of evaluations is also needed in other areas [42]. These include the proper identification and use of control groups; correlation of cognitive, attitudinal, and behavioral measures of change; assessing the possibility of underuse as a side effect of the program; and consideration of the rights of physicians as subjects in the study. Because the physician is the object of change, the physicians' behavior should be the unit of measure, not aggregate behavior which might obscure effects on individual physicians.

References

1. Fuchs, V.R., and J.P. Newhouse. National Bureau of Economic Research Conference on the Economics of Physician and Patient Behavior: The conference and unresolved problems. *J. Hum. Resour.* 1978; 13(suppl):1–18.

2. Roos, N.P. Hysterectomy: Variation in rates across small areas and across physicians' practices. *Am. J. Public Health.* 1984; 74:327–35.

3. Wennberg, J.E., K. McPherson, and P. Caper. Will payment based on diagnosis related groups control hospital costs? *N. Engl. J. Med.* 1984; 311:295–300.

4. Wennberg, J.E. Dealing with medical practice variations: A proposal for action. *Health Aff.* 1984; 3:6–32.

5. Wilensky, G.R., and L.F. Rossiter. The relative importance of physician-induced demand for medical care. *Milbank Mem. Fund Q.* 1983; 61:252–77.

6. Rossiter, L.F., and G.R. Wilensky. A reexamination of the use of physician services: The role of physician-initiated demand. *Inquiry.* 1983; 20:162–72.

7. Noren, J., T. Frazier, I. Altman, and J. DeLozier. Ambulatory medical care: A comparison of internists and family-general practitioners. *N. Engl. J. Med.* 1980; 302:11–16.

8. Fineberg, H.V., A.R. Funkhouser, and H. Marks. Variation in medical practice: A review of the literature. Presented at the Conference on Cost-Effective Medical Care: Implications of Variation in Medical Practice, Institute of Medicine, National Academy of Sciences, Washington, D.C., February 1983.

9. McDonald, C.J., S.L. Hui, D.M. Smith, et al. Reminders to physicians from an introspective computer medical record: A two-year randomized trial. *Ann. Intern. Med.* 1984; 100:130–38.

10. Naisbitt, J. *Megatrends.* New York: Warner Books, 1982; 17.

11. Eliot, T.S. The Rock. In *Collected Poems 1909–1962.* New York: Harcourt, Brace & World, 1963.

12. Johnson, A.N., and G.L. Appel. DRGs and hospital case records: Implications for Medicare case mix. *Inquiry.* 1984; 21:128–34.

13. Institute of Medicine. *Final Report: The Reliability of Medicare Hospital Discharge Records.* Washington, D.C.: Institute of Medicine, National Academy of Sciences, November 1977.

14. Roos, N.P., and L.L. Roos, Jr. Surgical rate variations: Do they reflect the health or socioeconomic characteristics of the populations? *Med. Care.* 1982; 20:945–58.

15. Bunker, J.P., L.L. Roos, Jr., J. Fowles, et al. Four information systems and routine monitoring. In Holland, W., ed. *Oxford Textbook of Public Health.* New York: Oxford University Press. In press.

16. See reference 2 above.

17. See reference 12 above.

18. Office of Technology Assessment. *Variations in Hospital Length of Stay: Their Relationship to Health Outcomes.* Washington, D.C.: Office of Technology Assessment, Congress of the United States, August 1983.

19. Lee, K., and A. Mills. *The Economics of Health in Developing Countries.* New York: Oxford University Press, 1983.

20. Newhouse, J.P., W.G. Manning, C.N. Morris, et al. Some interim results from a controlled trial of cost sharing in health insurance. *N. Engl. J. Med.* 1981; 305:1501–7.

21. Williams, S.V., J.M. Eisenberg, L.A. Pascale, and D.S. Kitz. Physicians' perceptions about unnecessary diagnostic testing. *Inquiry.* 1982; 19:363–70.

22. White, R.E., B.B. Quimby, B.J. Skipper, and G.D. Webster. Cost of resi-

dents' decisions on actual patients and in simulated encounters. *J. Med. Educ.* 1984; 59:834–35.

23. See reference 6 above.

24. Bailit, H.L., J.A. Balzer, and J. Clive. Evaluation of focused dental utilization review system. *Med. Care.* 1983; 21:473–85.

25. Elstein, A.S., M.M. Holmes, M.M. Ravitch, D.R. Romer, G.B. Holzman, and M.L. Rothert. Medical decisions in perspective: Applied research in cognitive psychology. *Perspect. Biol. Med.* 1983; 26:486–501.

26. Eisenberg, J.M. Sociological influences on decision making by clinicians. *Ann. Intern. Med.* 1979; 90:957–64.

27. Bailit, H.L., and J. Clive. The development of dental practice profiles. *Med. Care.* 1981; 19:30–46.

28. See reference 8 above.

29. Diehr, P. Small area statistics: Large statistical problems. *Am. J. Public Health.* 1984; 74:313–14.

30. Williams, R.L., and P.M. Chen. Controlling the rise in cesarean section rates by the dissemination of information from vital records. *Am. J. Public Health.* 1983; 73:863–67.

31. See reference 4 above.

32. Connor, M.J., and D. Gillings. An empiric study of ecological inference. *Am. J. Public Health.* 1984; 74:555–59.

33. Eisenberg, J.M. Modifying physician patterns of laboratory use. In Connelly, D.P., E.S. Benson, M.D. Burke, and D. Fenderson, eds. *Clinical Decisions and Laboratory Use.* Minneapolis: University of Minnesota Press, 1982; 145–58.

34. Whiting-O'Keefe, Q.E., C. Henke, and D.W. Simborg. Choosing the correct unit of analysis in medical care experiments. *Med. Care.* 1984; 22:1101–14.

35. See reference 33 above.

36. See reference 24 above.

37. Eisenberg, J.M., and S.V. Williams. The usefulness of the proportion of tests with normal results in diagnostic services utilization review. *Clin. Chem.* 1983; 29:2111–13.

38. Brook, R.H., and K.N. Lohr. Second opinion programs: Beyond cost-benefit analyses. *Med. Care.* 1982; 20:1–2.

39. Perkoff, G.T. Economic versus professional incentives for cost control. *N. Engl. J. Med.* 1982; 307:1399–1401.

40. Schroeder, S.A., L.P. Myers, S.J. McPhee, et al. The failure of physician education as a cost containment strategy: Report of a prospective controlled trial at a university hospital. *J.A.M.A.* 1984; 252:225–30.

41. Brook, R.H., J.E. Ware, W.H. Rogers, et al. Does free care improve adults' health? Results from a randomized controlled trial. *N. Engl. J. Med.* 1983; 309:1426–34.

42. See reference 33 above.

9

Why Should We Care?

The challenges for health services researchers who investigate the factors that influence providers' utilization of services offer exciting opportunities to contribute to an understanding of how medical care is provided and ways in which it can be improved. As new ways of organizing and paying for medical care are introduced, the research community should envision them as opportunities, as experiments in nature. These new programs provide the researcher with laboratories in which to test hypotheses about how doctors and hospitals respond to new economics or sociology of medical practice.

Much of the research about physicians' practice patterns has dealt with rates of surgery or use of diagnostic tests. The reason for this is not necessarily because these are the most important decisions that doctors make, but rather because at least some data are available about these decisions. Explicit measures of surgery and laboratory test use can be defined. The indications for their use may be difficult to define, but progress has been made. Also, evidence has shown overuse of both these medical care services, and reasonably large numbers of these services are provided per doctor so that the provider can be considered as the unit of statistical analysis. In addition, information systems are available that provide data about the utilization rates of these services. Efforts have been made to change practice patterns in these areas and have shown some methods to be potentially more effective than others. It has become clear that research in this area is feasible. For all the methodological challenges in this area of health services research, the last 15 years have given cause for optimism. There is reason to believe that much can be learned from utilization studies about the factors that influence medical decision making and how to manipulate these factors to change practice patterns. In addition, the ultimate goal of more value for resources spent on medical care appears now to be one that can be accomplished.

The implications of research on physician behavior and the factors that influence medical decision making are increasingly pertinent as the constraints on the resources available for medical care become more apparent. As policy makers and national leaders in medicine seek ways to ensure that the most value can be obtained for the money spent on medical care and as efforts to improve the care that is delivered by individual physicians continue, it becomes critical to understand the underpinnings of physician practice patterns.

The failure of Professional Standards Review Organizations was due in large measure to the lack of effective instruments to change physicians [1]. The idea that penalties to hospitals for overutilization would trickle down to effective interventions at the physicians' level was naive. Today, in the face of the economic pressures of reimbursement based on diagnosis related groups, hospital administrators are again searching for ways to influence the doctors on their staffs. Without financial incentives for the doctor, they will need to rely on other proven ways of changing physicians' practice, particularly individualized feedback from clinical leaders and participation by physicians in cost-containment efforts. Even without the financial incentive of per-case reimbursement for physicians, some hospitals may be able to translate the hospital's economic incentives into incentives for physicians. New hospital-physician alliances should provide a forum for seeking cost-effective medical practices. The success of health maintenance organizations in reducing hospitalization, particularly in comparison to that of individual practice associations, demonstrates the powerful influence of organizational ethos and peer pressure.

Despite physicians' desires to act as their patients' perfect agents, seeking only to maximize the patients' own preferred outcomes, physicians are buffeted by forces outside the doctor-patient encounter. One of the most malleable of these influences is the schedule of fees for services. The present economic incentives that encourage procedures and penalize the interpersonal aspects of practice leave few physicians untouched. As expected, physicians may read these signals as an indication of the kind of medicine that society wants. Physicians will deliver that which society rewards, constrained, it is hoped, by personal and professional ethics and concern for the patient's well-being. Despite the importance of non-economic influences on physicians' practice patterns, the economic desires of physicians could be harnessed to promote, rather than obstruct, cost-effective medical care if new payment systems were designed to shape practice patterns.

The mere presence of variation among providers should not necessarily be bemoaned. Because patients' preferences are clearly not all the same, it may be that variation serves at least one useful purpose: it enables patients to seek care from doctors whose practice styles are consistent with their preferences. Given these differences in public desires and values, we would not want to minimize variation among providers below some minimum level. Although we do not know what the minimum level of variation might be for different services, the evaluation of reasonable levels of variation would make interesting grist for the researcher's mill.

Further policy implications of the research on physicians' utilization relate to the need for development and evaluation of data systems. The emergence of valid data bases could provide managers of the medical care enterprise with the information they need to feed back to physicians, to target programs to change physicians' behavior, to assess physicians' responses to interventions, and to evalute long-term changes in practice patterns. Although recent Congressional interest in disclosing Medicare data which is hospital- and physician-specific suggests a commitment to evaluation of utilization data as a way of determining differences in the cost and quality of medical care, this action may be premature. Without antecedent support of the research needed to validate the data and evaluate their meaning with regard to cost and quality, the wholesale release of claims data could be more misleading than informative. The complex interaction of factors that influence medical decision making and the methodological challenges of research in this area will require the contribution of health service researchers from a number of fields, including clinical practice, medical decision making, clinical epidemiology, economics, statistics, and sociology.

The way in which physicians decide to practice medicine is obviously influenced by a multitude of factors. None is sufficient alone to explain medical decision making, but the "black box" has been partly opened by research on physicians' behavior, most of which is less than 15 years old. The size of the health care engine may be determined by decisions about capital expenditures and the acquisition of new technology. Still, the central role of the physician in determining the speed with which the health care engine is driven makes understanding medical decision making central to ensuring that limited resources are used efficiently.

Reference

1. Eisenberg, J.M., and A.J. Rosoff. Physician responsibility for the cost of unnecessary medical services. *N. Engl. J. Med.* 1978; 299:76–80.

Bibliography

Abel-Smith, B. *Cost Containment in Health Care: A Study of 12 European Countries, 1977–1983*. London: Bedford Square Press of the National Council for Voluntary Organizations, 1984. Occasional Papers on Social Administration, No. 73.

Abrams, H.L. The 'overutilization' of x-rays. *N. Engl. J. Med.* 1979; 300:1213–16.

Adler, N.E., and A. Milstein. Evaluating the impact of physician peer review: Factors associated with successful PSROs. *Am. J. Public Health.* 1983; 73:1182–85.

Altman, L.K. Prank punishes young surgeons. *New York Times.* 1984 September 4.

Anderson, J.G., and S.J. Jay. Utilization of computers in clinical practice: The role of physician networks—preliminary communication. *J. R. Soc. Med.* 1983; 76:45–52.

Anderson, O.W., and M.C. Shields. Quality measurement and control in physician decision making: State of the art. *Health Serv. Res.* 1982; 17:125–55.

Applegate, W.B., M.D. Bennett, L. Chilton. B.J. Skipper, and R.E. White. Impact of a cost containment educational program on housestaff ambulatory clinic charges. *Med. Care.* 1983; 21:486–96.

Arrow, K.J. Uncertainty and the welfare economics of medical care. *Am. Econ. Rev.* 1963; 53:941–73.

Avorn, J., M. Chen, and R. Hartley. Scientific versus commercial sources of influence on the prescribing behavior of physicians. *Am. J. Med.* 1982; 73:4–8.

Avorn, J., and S.B. Soumerai. A new approach to reducing suboptimal drug use. *J.A.M.A.* 1983; 250:1752–53.

Avorn, J., and S.B. Soumerai. Improving drug-therapy decisions through educational outreach: A randomized controlled trial of academically based 'detailing.' *N. Engl. J. Med.* 1983; 308:1457–63.

Bailey, R.M. *Clinical Laboratories and the Practice of Medicine.* Berkeley, Calif.: McCutchan Publishing Corp., 1979.

Bailit, H.L., J.A. Balzer, and J. Clive. Evaluation of focused dental utilization review system. *Med. Care.* 1983; 21:473–85.

Bailit, H.L., and J. Clive. The development of dental practice profiles. *Med. Care.* 1981; 19:30–46.

Barr, J.K., and M.K. Steinberg. Professional participation in organizational decision making: Physicians in HMOs. *J. Community Health.* 1983; 8:160–73.

Becker, E.R., and F.A. Sloan. Utilization of hospital services: The roles of teaching, case mix, and reimbursement. *Inquiry.* 1983; 20:248–57.

Becker, M.H. Sociometric location and innovativeness: Reformulation and extension of the diffusion model. *Am. Sociol. Rev.* 1970; 35:267–82.

Berbatis, C.G., M.J. Maher, R.J. Plumridge, J.U. Stoelwinder, and S.R. Zubrick. Impact of a drug bulletin on prescribing oral analgesics in a teaching hospital. *Am. J. Hosp. Pharm.* 1982; 38:98–100.

Berger, J.D. Physician involvement in hospital cost control. *Hosp. Forum.* 1983; 26:17–21.

Berner, E.S., L.R. Coulson, and B.P. Schmitt. A method to determine attitudes of faculty members toward use of laboratory tests. *J. Med. Educ.* 1985; 60:374–78.

Berry, C., P.J. Held, B. Kehrer, L. Marheim, and U. Reinhardt. Canadian physicians' supply response to Universal Health Insurance: The first years in Quebec (preliminary results). In Gabel, J.R., J. Taylor, N.T. Greenspan, and M. Blaxall, eds. *Physicians and Financial Incentives.* Washington, D.C.: U.S. Government Printing Office, 1980; 57–59.

Bloomgarden, Z., and V.W. Sidel. Evaluation of utilization of laboratory tests in a hospital emergency room. *Am. J. Public Health.* 1980; 70:525–28.

Bloor, M. Bishop Berkeley and the adenotonsillectomy enigma: An exploration of variation in the social construction of medical disposals. *Sociology.* 1976; 10:43–61.

Bloor, M.J., G.A. Venters, and M.L. Samphier. Geographical variation in the incidence of operations on the tonsils and adenoids: An epidemiological and sociological investigation. Part I. *J. Laryngol. Otol.* 1978; 92:791–801.

Bloor, M.J., G.A. Venters, and M.L. Samphier. Geographical variation in the incidence of operations on the tonsils and adenoids: An epidemiological and sociological investigation. Part II. *J. Laryngol. Otol.* 1978; 92:883–95.

Blumberg, M.S. Regional differences in hospital use standardized by reported morbidity. *Med. Care.* 1982; 20:931–44.

Boardman, A.E., B. Dowd, J.M. Eisenberg, et al. A model of physicians' practice attributes determination. *J. Health Econ.* 1984; 2:259–68.

Boice, J.L., and M. McGregor. Effect of residents' use of laboratory tests on hospital costs. *J. Med. Educ.* 1983; 58:61–64.

Boyd, J.C., D.E. Bruns, B.W. Renoe, J. Savory, and M.R. Witts. Medical education in laboratory testing: An approach incorporating the student's own laboratory results. *Am. J. Clin. Pathol.* 1983; 79:211–16.

Brook, R.H., and K.N. Lohr. Second opinion programs: Beyond cost-benefit analyses. *Med. Care.* 1982; 20:1–2.

Brook, R.H., J.E. Ware, W.H. Rogers, et al. Does free care improve adults' health? Results from a randomized controlled trial. *N. Engl. J. Med.* 1983; 309:1426–34.

Brook, R.H., and K.N. Williams. Effect of medical care review on the use of injections: A study of the New Mexico Experimental Medical Care Review Organization. *Ann. Intern. Med.* 1976; 85:509–15.

Brook, R.H., K.N. Williams, and J.E. Rolph. Controlling the use and cost of medical services: The New Mexico Experimental Medical Care Review Organization—a four year case study. *Med. Care.* 1978; 16(suppl):1–76.

Brook, R.H., K.N. Williams, and J.E. Rolph. Use, costs, and quality of medical services: Impact of the New Mexico Peer Review System—A 1971–1975 study. *Ann. Intern. Med.* 1978; 89:256–63.

Buck, C.R., Jr., and K.L. White. Peer review: Impact of a system based on billings claims. *N. Engl. J. Med.* 1974; 291:877–83.

Bunker, J.P. Surgical manpower: A comparison of operations and surgeons in the United States and in England and Wales. *N. Engl. J. Med.* 1970; 282:135–44.

Bunker, J.P. When doctors disagree. *N.Y. Rev. Books.* 1985; 32(7):8–12.

Bunker, J.P., H.S. Luft, and A. Enthoven. Should surgery be regionalized? *Surg. Clin. No. Am.* 1982; 62:657–68.

Bunker, J.P., L.L. Roos, J. Fowles, et al. Four information systems and routine monitoring. In Holland, W., ed. *Oxford Textbook of Public Health.* New York: Oxford University Press. In press.

Cageorge, S.M., and L.L. Roos. When surgical rates change: Workload and turnover in Manitoba, 1974–1978. *Med. Care.* 1984; 22:890–900.

Campbell, D.M. Why do physicians in neonatal care units differ in their admission thresholds? *Soc. Sci. Med.* 1984; 18:365–74.

Caper, P., and M. Zubkoff. Managing medical costs through small area analysis. *Bus. Health.* 1984 September 20: 20–25.

Cebul, R.D. "A look at the chief complaints" revisited. *Med. Decis. Making.* 1984; 4:271–83.

Cebul, R.D., and L.H. Beck. *Teaching Clinical Decision Making.* New York: Praeger Publishing, 1986.

Cebul, R.D., L.H. Beck, J.G. Carroll, et al. A course in clinical decision making adaptable to different audiences. *Med. Decis. Making.* 1984; 4:285–96.

Chassin, M.R. *Variations in Hospital Length of Stay: Their Relationship to Health Outcomes.* Washington, D.C.: Office of Technology Assessment, Congress of the United States, August 1983.

Check, W.A. How to affect antibiotic prescribing practices. *J.A.M.A.* 1980; 244:2594–95.

Childs, A.W., and E.D. Hunter. Non-medical factors influencing use of diagnostic x-rays by physicians. *Med. Care.* 1972; 10:323–35.

Chokshi, A.B., H.S. Friedman, M. Malach, B.C. Vasvada, and S.J. Bleicher. Impact of peer review in reduction of permanent pacemaker implantations. *J.A.M.A.* 1981; 240:754–57.

Christensen-Szalanski, J.J.J. Discount functions and the measurement of patient values: Women's decisions during childbirth. *Med. Decis. Making.* 1984; 4:47–48.

Chu, R.C., S.V. Williams, and J.M. Eisenberg. The characteristics of stat laboratory tests. *Arch. Pathol. Lab. Med.* 1982; 106:662–65.

Cohen, D.I., P. Jones, B. Littenberg, and D. Neuhauser. Does cost information availability reduce physician test usage? A randomized clinical trial with unexpected findings. *Med. Care.* 1982; 20:286–92.

Cohen, D.I., B. Littenberg, C. Wetzel, and D. Neuhauser. Improving physician compliance with preventive medicine guidelines. *Med. Care.* 1982; 20:1040–45.

Coleman, J.S., E. Katz, and H. Menzel. *Medical Innovation: A Diffusion Study.* New York: Bobbs-Merrill, 1966.

Coleman, J.S., H. Menzel, and E. Katz. Social process in physicians' adoption of a new drug. *J. Chronic Dis.* 1959; 9:1–9.

Collen, M.F. *Utilization of Diagnostic X-Ray Examinations.* Washington, D.C.: National Center for Devices and Radiological Health, Food and Drug Administration, Public Health Service, August 1983.

Connell, F.A., L.A. Blide, and M.A. Hanken. Clinical correlates of small area variation in population based admission rates for diabetes. *Med. Care.* 1984; 22:939–49.

Connell, F.A., R.W. Day, and J.P. LoGerfo. Hospitalization of Medicaid children: Analysis of small area variations in admission rates. *Am. J. Public Health.* 1981; 71:606–13.

Connor, M.J., and D. Gillings. An empiric study of ecological inference. *Am. J. Public Health.* 1984; 74:555–59.

Craig, W.A., S.J. Ulman, W.R. Shaw, V. Ramgopal, L.L. Eagan, and E.T. Leopold. Hospital use of antimicrobial drugs: Survey at 19 hospitals and results of antimicrobial control programs. *Ann. Intern. Med.* 1978; 89:739–95.

Cummings, K.M., K.B. Frisof, M.J. Long, and G. Krynkiewich. The effect of price information on physicians' test ordering behavior: Ordering of diagnostic tests. *Med. Care.* 1982; 20:293.

Daniels, M., and S.A. Schroeder. Variation among physicians in use of laboratory tests: II. Relation to clinical productivity and outcomes of care. *Med. Care.* 1977; 15:482–87.

Danzon, P.M. *Economic Factors in the Use of Laboratory Tests by Office-Based Physicians.* Santa Monica, Calif: Rand Corp., August 1982. Rand Corp. Pub. R–2525–1–HCFA.

Danzon, P.M., W.G. Manning, and M.S. Marquis. *Factors Affecting Laboratory*

Test Use and Price. Santa Monica, Calif.; Rand Corp., January 1983. Rand Corp. Pub. R–2987–HCFA.

Danzon, P.M., W.G. Manning, and M.S. Marquis. Factors influencing laboratory test use and prices. *Health Care Financing Rev.* 1984; 5:23–32.

Davis, D., R.B. Haynes, L. Chambers, V.R. Neufield, A. McKibbon, and P. Tugwell. The impact of CME: A methodological review of the continuing medical education literature. *Eval. Health Prof.* 1984; 7:251–83.

DesHarnais, S., N.M. Kibe, and S. Barbus. Blue Cross and Blue Shield of Michigan Hospital Laboratory On-Site Review Project. *Inquiry.* 1983; 20:328–33.

Devitt, J.E., and M.R. Ironside. Can patient care audit change doctor performance? *J. Med. Educ.* 1975; 50:1122–23.

Diehr, P. Small area statistics: Large statistical problems. *Am. J. Public Health.* 1984; 74:313–14.

Dietrich, A.J., and H. Goldberg. Preventive content of adult primary care: Do generalists and subspecialists differ? *Am. J. Public Health.* 1984; 74:223–27.

Dixon, R.H., and J. Laszlo. Utilization of clinical chemistry services by medical house staff: An analysis. *Arch. Intern. Med.* 1974; 134:1064–67.

Dorsey, J.L. Use of diagnostic resources in health maintenance organizations and fee-for-service practice settings. *Arch. Intern. Med.* 1983; 143:1863–65.

Duke Law Project. The medical malpractice threat: A study of defensive medicine. *Duke Law J.* 1971; 939–72.

Dunlop, D.M., R.S. Inch, and J. Paul. A survey of prescribing in Scotland in 1951. *Br. Med. J.* 1953; 1:694–97.

Durbin, W.A., Jr., B. Lapidas, and D.A. Goldmann. Improved antibiotic usage following introduction of a novel prescription system. *J.A.M.A.* 1981; 246:1796–1800.

Eastaugh, S.R. Cost of elective surgery and utilization of ancillary services in teaching hospitals. *Health Serv. Res.* 1979; 14:290–308.

Eddy, D.M. Clinical policies and the quality of clinical practice. *N. Engl. J. Med.* 1982; 307:343–47.

Eddy, D.M. Variations in physician practice: The role of uncertainty. *Health Aff.* 1984; 3:74–89.

Eisenberg, J.M. An educational program to modify laboratory use by house staff. *J. Med. Educ.* 1977; 52:578–81.

Eisenberg, J.M. Modifying physicians' patterns of laboratory use. In Connelly, D.P., E.S. Benson, M.D. Burke, and D. Fenderson, eds. *Clinical Decisions and Laboratory Use.* Minneapolis: University of Minneapolis Press, 1982; 145–58.

Eisenberg, J.M. Physician utilization: The state of research about physicians' practice patterns. *Med. Care.* 1985; 23:461–83.

Eisenberg, J.M. Sociological influences on decision making by clinicians. *Ann. Intern. Med.* 1979; 90:957–64.

Eisenberg, J.M. The internist as gatekeeper. *Ann. Intern. Med.* 1985; 102:537–43.

Eisenberg, J.M. The use of ancillary services: A role for utilization review? *Med. Care.* 1982; 20:849–61.

Eisenberg, J.M., and J.C. Hershey. Derived thresholds: Determining the diagnostic probabilities at which clinicians initiate testing and treatment. *Med. Decis. Making.* 1983; 3:155–68.

Eisenberg, J.M., D.S. Kitz, and R.A. Webber. Development of attitudes about sharing decision making: A comparison of medical and surgical residents. *J. Health Soc. Behav.* 1983; 24:85–90.

Eisenberg, J.M., and D. Nicklin. Use of diagnostic services by physicians in community practice. *Med. Care.* 1981; 19:297–309.

Eisenberg, J.M., and A.J. Rosoff. Physician responsibility for the cost of unnecessary medical service. *N. Engl. J. Med.* 1978; 299:76–80.

Eisenberg, J.M., and S.V. Williams. Cost containment and changing physicians' practice behavior: Can the fox learn to guard the chicken coop? *J.A.M.A.* 1981; 246:2195–2201.

Eisenberg, J.M., and S.V. Williams. The usefulness of the proportion of tests with normal results in diagnostic services utilization review. *Clin. Chem.* 1983; 29:2111–13.

Eisenberg, J.M., S.V. Williams, L. Garner, R. Viale, and H. Smits. Computer-based audit to detect and correct overutilization of laboratory tests. *Med. Care.* 1977; 15:915–21.

Eliot, T.S. The Rock. *In Collected Poems: 1909–1962.* New York: Harcourt, Brace and World, 1963.

Ellwood, P.M. When MDs meet DRGs. *Hospitals.* 1983; 57(Dec. 16):62–66.

Elstein, A.S., M.M. Holmes, M.M. Ravitch, D.R. Romer, G.B. Holzman, and M.L. Rothert. Medical decisions in perspective: Applied research in cognitive psychology. *Perspect. Biol. Med.* 1983; 26:486–501.

Ende, J. Feedback in clinical medical education. *J.A.M.A.* 1983; 250:777–81.

Epstein, A.M., C.B. Begg, and B.J. McNeil. The effects of group size on test ordering for hypertensive patients. *N. Engl. J. Med.* 1983; 309:464–68.

Epstein, A.M., C.B. Begg, and B.J. McNeil. The effects of physician training and personality on test ordering for ambulatory patients. *Am. J. Public Health.* 1984; 74:1271–73.

Epstein, A.M., R.M. Hartley, J.R. Charlton, et al. A comparison of ambulatory test ordering for hypertensive patients in the United States and England. *J.A.M.A.* 1984; 252:1723–26.

Epstein, A.M., S.J. Krock, and B.J. McNeil. Office laboratory tests: Perceptions of profitability. *Med. Care.* 1984; 22:160–66.

Ernst, R. Ancillary production and the size of physicians' practice. *Inquiry.* 1976; 13:371–81.

Estes, E.H., Jr. The behavior of health professionals: Impact on cost and quality of care. *Duke Univ. Med. Cent. Perspect.* 1983; 3:7–13.

Evans, R.C. Supplier-induced demand: Some empirical evidence and implications. In Perlman, M., ed. *The Economics of Health and Medical Care.* New York: John Wiley & Sons, 1974.

Evans, R.W. Health care technology and the inevitability of resource allocation and rationing decisions: Part I. *J.A.M.A.* 1983; 249:2047–53.

Everett, G.D., P.F. Chang, C.S. de Blois, and T.D. Holets. A comparative study of laboratory utilization behavior on "on-service" and "off-service" housestaff physicians. *Med. Care.* 1983; 21:1187–91.

Everett, G.D., C.S. de Blois, and P.F. Chang. Impact of medical school laboratory courses and physician attitude on test use by house staff. *J. Med. Educ.* 1983; 58:736–38.

Everett, G.D., C.S. de Blois, P.F. Chang, and T.D.Holets. Effect of cost education, cost audits, and faculty chart review on the use of laboratory services. *Arch. Intern. Med.* 1983; 143:942–44.

Feldman, R., R. Goldfarb, J. Rafferty, and M.Goldfarb. Physician choice of patient load and mode of treatment. *Atl. Econ. J.* 1981; 9:69–78.

Feldstein, M.S. The rising price of physicians' services. *Rev. Stat.* 1970; 52:121–33.

Ferster, C.B., and B.F. Skinner. *Schedules of Reinforcement.* New York: Appleton-Century-Crofts, 1957.

Fineberg, H.V., A.R. Funkhouser, and H. Marks. Variation in medical practice: A review of the literature. Presented at the Conference on Cost-Effective Medical Care: Implications of Variation in Medical Practice, Institute of Medicine, National Academy of Sciences, Washington, D.C., February 1983.

Fishbane, M., and B. Starfield. Child health care in the United States: A comparison of pediatricians and general practitioners. *N. Engl. J. Med.* 1981; 305:552–56.

Flood, A.B., W.R. Scott, W. Ewy, and W.H. Forrest, Jr. Effectiveness in professional organizations: The impact of surgeons and surgical staff organizations on the quality of care in hospitals. *Health Serv. Res.* 1982; 17:341–66.

Forrest, J.B., W.P. Ritchie, M. Hudson, and J.F. Harlan. Cost containment through cost awareness: A strategy that failed. *Surgery.* 1981; 90:154–58.

Fowkes, F.G.R., L.A. Williams, B.R.B. Cooke, R.C. Evans, S.H. Gehlbach, and C.J. Roberts. Implementation of guidelines for the use of skull radiographs in patients with head injuries. *Lancet.* 1984; 2:795–96.

Freeborn, D.K., D. Baer, M.R. Greenlick, and J.W. Bailey. Determinants of medical care utilization: Physicians' use of laboratory services. *Am. J. Public Health.* 1972; 62:846–53.

Freeman, R.A. Cost containment. *J. Med. Educ.* 1976; 51:157–58.

Freidson, E. *Profession of Medicine: A Study of the Sociology of Applied Knowledge.* New York: Dodd, Mead & Co., 1970.

Freymann, J.G. Teaching economic reality to medical students. *Bus. Health.* 1985; (April):14–18.

Fried, C. Rights and health care: Beyond equity and efficiency. *N. Engl. J. Med.* 1975; 293:241–45.

Fuchs, V.R. The supply of surgeons and the demand for operations. *J. Hum. Resour.* 1978; 13(suppl):35–56.

Fuchs, V.R. *Who Shall Live? Health, Economics and Social Change.* New York: Basic Books, 1974.

Fuchs, V.R., and M.J. Kramer. *Determinants of Expenditures for Physicians' Services in the United States 1948–68.* Washington, D.C.: National Center for Health

Services Research and Development, Department of Health Education and Welfare, December 1972; 1–63. DHEW publication no. (HSM) 73–3013.

Fuchs, V.R., and J.P. Newhouse. National Bureau of Economic Research Conference on the economics of physician and patient behavior: The conference and unresolved problems. *J. Hum. Resour.* 1978; 13(suppl):1–18.

Gabel, J.R., and T.H. Rice. Reducing public expenditures for physician services: The price of paying less. *J. Health Polit. Policy Law.* 1985; 9:595–609.

Garber, A.M., V.R. Fuchs, and J.F. Silverman. Case mix, cost and outcomes. *N. Engl. J. Med.* 1984; 310:1231–37.

Garg, M.L., W.A. Gliebe, and M.B. Elkhatib. The extent of defensive medicine: Some empirical evidence. *Leg. Aspects Med. Practice.* 1978; 6:25–29.

Geertsma, R.H., R.C. Parker, Jr., and S.K. Whitbourne. How physicians view the process of change in their practice behavior. *J. Med. Educ.* 1982; 57:752–61.

Gehlbach, S.H., W.E. Wilkinson, W.E. Hammond, et al. Improving drug prescribing in a primary care practice. *Med. Care.* 1984; 22:193–201.

Gertman, P.M., A.C. Monheit, J.J. Anderson, J.B. Eagle, and D.K. Levenson. Utilization review in the United States: Results from a 1976–1977 national survey of hospitals. *Med. Care.* 1979; 17(suppl):1–148.

Gertman, P.M., and J.D. Restuccia. The appropriateness evaluation protocol: A technique for assessing unnecessary days of hospital care. *Med. Care.* 1981; 19:855–71.

Gibson, R.M., D.R. Waldo, and K.R. Levit. National health expenditures, 1982. *Health Care Financing Rev.* 1983; 5:1–33.

Gold, M. Effects of hospital-based primary care setting on internists' treatment of primary care episodes. *Health Serv. Res.* 1981; 16:383–405.

Gold, M., and M. Greenlick. Effect of hospital-based primary care setting on internists' use of inpatient hospital resources. *Med. Care.* 1981; 19:160–71.

Goldfarb, M.G., M.C. Hornbrook, and C.S. Higgins. Determinants of hospital use: A cross-diagnostic analysis. *Med. Care.* 1983; 21:48–66.

Goodspeed, R., F. Davidoff, M. Testa, and J. Clive. "Little ticket" laboratory tests: Differential effect of probabilistic vs. cost-control curriculum on ordering rates [Abstract]. *Clin. Res.* 1985; 33:721A.

Gornick, M. Medicare patients: Geographic differences in hospital discharge rates and multiple stays. *Soc. Secur. Bull.* 1977; (June):1–20.

Greenland, P., A.I. Mushlin, and P.F. Griner. Discrepancies between knowledge and use of diagnostic studies in asymptomatic patients. *J. Med. Educ.* 1979; 54:863–69.

Greenwald, H.P., M.L. Peterson, L.P. Garrison, et al. Interspecialty variation in office-based care. *Med. Care.* 1984; 22:14–29.

Greer, A.L. Advances in the study of diffusion of innovation in health care organizations. *Milbank Mem. Fund Q.* 1977; 55:505–62.

Greer, A.L. Medical technology and professional dominance theory. *Soc. Sci. Med.* 1984; 10:809–17.

Griner, P.F. Use of laboratory tests in a teaching hospital: Long-term trends—reductions in use and relative cost. *Ann. Intern. Med.* 1979; 90:243–48.

Griner, P.F., and R.J. Glaser. Misuse of laboratory tests and diagnostic procedures. *N. Engl. J. Med.* 1982; 307:1336–39.

Grivell, A.R., H.J. Forgie, C.J. Fraser, and M.N. Berry. Effect of feedback to clinical staff of information on clinical biochemistry requesting patterns. *Clin. Chem.* 1981; 27:1717–20.

Grossman, R.M. A review of physician cost-containment strategies for laboratory testing. *Med. Care.* 1983; 21:783–802.

Gryskiewicz, J.M., and D.E. Detmer. Waste not, want not: Use of blood in elective operations—improved utilization of blood by use of blood-ordering protocols and the type and screen. *Curr. Surg.* 1983; 40:371–77.

Hadley, J. Physician participation in Medicaid: Evidence from California. *Health Serv. Res.* 1979; 14:266–80.

Hadsall, R.S., R.A. Freeman, and G.J. Norwood. Factors related to the prescribing of selected psychotropic drugs by primary care physicians. *Soc. Sci. Med.* 1982; 16:1747–56.

Hale, F.A., K.C. Stone, D.J. Serbert, and E.C. Nelson. A clinical cost-consciousness learning packet for community-based clerkships. *Fam. Med.* 1984; 16:131–33.

Hall, D. Prescribing as social exchange. In Mapes, R., ed. *Prescribing Practice and Drug Usage.* London: Croom Helm, 1980; 39–57.

Hall, F.M. Overutilization of radiological examinations. *Radiology.* 1976; 120:443–48.

Hardin, G. The tragedy of the commons. *Science.* 1968; 162:1243–48.

Hardwick, D.F., P. Vertinsky, R.T. Barth, V.F. Mitchell, M. Bernstein, and I. Vertinsky. Clinical styles and motivation: A study of laboratory test use. *Med. Care.* 1975; 13:397–408.

Hartzema, A.G., and D.B. Christensen. Nonmedical factors associated with the prescribing volume among family practitioners in an HMO. *Med. Care.* 1983; 21:990–1000.

Hayes, L.F. Defensive medicine: The incorrect solution. *Mich. Med.* 1977; 76:267–68.

Heath, D.A., R. Hoffenberg, J.M. Bishop, M.J. Kendall, and O.L. Wade. Medical audits. *J. R. Coll. Phys.* 1980; 14:200–201.

Hemenway, D., and D. Fallon. Testing for physician-induced demand with hypothetical cases. *Med. Care.* 1985; 23:344–49.

Hershey, N. The defensive practice of medicine: Myth or reality. *Milbank Mem. Fund Q.* 1972; 50:69–98.

Heyssel, R.M., J.R. Gaintner, I.W. Kues, A.A. Jones, and S.H. Lipstein. Decentralized management in a teaching hospital. *N. Engl. J. Med.* 1984; 310:1477–80.

Hiatt, H.H. Protecting the medical commons: Who is responsible? *N. Engl. J. Med.* 1975; 293:235–41.

Hillman, R.S., S. Helbig, S. Howes, J. Hayes, D.M. Meyer, and J.R. McArthur.

The effect of an educational program on transfusion practices in a regional blood program. *Transfusion.* 1979; 19:153–57.

Hirsh, H.L., and T.S. Dickey. Defensive medicine as a basis for malpractice liability. *Trans. Stud. Coll. Physicians Phila.* 1983; 5:98–107.

Hlatky, M.A., K.L. Lee, E.H. Botvinich, and B.H. Brundage. Diagnostic test use in different practice settings: A controlled comparison. *Arch. Intern. Med.* 1983; 143:1886–89.

Hoey, J., J.M. Eisenberg, W.O. Spitzer, and D. Thomas. Physician sensitivity to the price of diagnostic tests: A U.S.–Canadian analysis. *Med. Care.* 1982; 20:302–7.

Hooper, E.M., L.M. Comstock, J.M. Goodwin, and J.S. Goodwin. Patient characteristics that influence physician behavior. *Med. Care.* 1982; 20:630–38.

Hornbrook, M.C., and M.G. Goldfarb. A partial test of a hospital behavioral model. *Soc. Sci. Med.* 1983; 17:667–80.

Hughes, R.A., P.M. Gertman, J.J. Anderson, et al. The Ancillary Services Review Program in Massachusetts: Experience of the 1982 pilot project. *J.A.M.A.* 1984; 252:1727–32.

Hulka, B., and J. Wheat. Patterns of utilization: The patient perspective. *Med. Care.* 1985; 23:438–60.

Hunt, D.D. Effects of incentives on economic behavior and productivity of psychiatric residents. *J. Psychiatr. Educ.* 1980; 4:4–13.

Institute of Medicine. *Institute of Medicine Final Report: The Reliability of Medicare Hospital Discharge Records.* Washington, D.C.: Institute of Medicine, National Academy of Sciences, November 1977.

Johns, R.J., and B.I. Blum. The use of clinical information systems to control cost as well as to improve care. *Trans. Am. Clin. Climatol. Assoc.* 1979; 90:140–42.

Johnson, A.N., and G.L. Appel. DRGs and hospital case records: Implications for Medicare case mix. *Inquiry.* 1984; 21:128–34.

Johnson, M.W., W.E. Mitch, A.H. Heller, and R. Spector. The impact of an educational program on gentamicin use in a teaching hospital. *Am. J. Med.* 1982; 73:9–14.

Jones, K.R. The influence of the attending physician on indirect graduate medical education costs. *J. Med. Educ.* 1984; 59:789–98.

Kaluzny, A.D. Innovation in health system: A selective review of system characteristics and empirical research. In Abernathy, W.J., A. Sheldon, and C.K. Prahalad, eds. *The Management of Health Care.* Cambridge, Mass.: Ballinger Publishing Co., 1974; 67–68.

Kaluzny, A.D., J.E. Veney, and J.T. Gentry. Innovation of health services: A comparative study of hospitals and health departments. *Milbank Mem. Fund Q.* 1974; 52:51–82.

Kassenbaum, D.G. Teaching laboratory test use. *J. Med. Educ.* 1985; 60:420–21.

Knapp, D.E., D.A. Knapp, M.K. Speedie, D.M. Yaeger, and C.L. Baker. Relationship of inappropriate drug prescribing to increased length of hospital stay. *Am. J. Hosp. Pharm.* 1979; 36:1334–37.

Koepsell, T.D., A.L. Gurtel, P.H. Diehr, et al. The Seattle evaluation of computerized drug profiles: Effects on prescribing practices and resource use. *Am. J. Public Health.* 1983; 73:850–55.

Lawrence, P.R., and J.W. Lorsch. *Organization and Environment: Managing Differentiation and Integration.* Cambridge, Mass.: Division of Research, Graduate School of Business Administration, Harvard University Press, 1967.

Lee, J.A. Prescribing and other aspects of general practice in three towns. *Proc. R. Soc. Med.* 1964; 57:1041–43.

Lee, J.A., P.A. Draper, and M. Weatherall. Prescribing in three English towns. *Milbank Mem. Fund Q.* 1965; 43:285–90.

Lee, K., and A. Mills. *The Economics of Health in Developing Countries.* New York: Oxford University Press, 1983.

Lewin, K. Group decision and social change. In Newcomb, T.M., and E.L. Hantley, eds. *Readings in Social Psychology.* New York: Holt, Rinehart and Winston, 1958.

Linn, L.S., J. Yager, B.D. Leake, et al. Differences in the numbers and costs of tests ordered by internists, family physicians and psychiatrists. *Inquiry.* 1984; 21:266–75.

Lion, J. Case-mix differences among ambulatory patients seen by internists in various settings. *Health Serv. Res.* 1981; 16:407–13.

Lipp, C.S. Peer review experiment succeeds in Delaware. *Bus. Health.* 1984; 1(6):21–24.

LoGerfo, J.P. Organizational and financial influences on patterns of surgical care. *Surg. Clin. North Am.* 1982; 62:677–84.

Long, M.J., K.M. Cummings, and K.B. Frisof. The role of perceived price in physicians' demand for diagnostic tests. *Med. Care.* 1983; 21:243–50.

Luft, H.S. How do health-maintenance organizations achieve their ""savings"? *N. Engl. J. Med.* 1978; 298:1336–43.

Luft, H.S. Variations in clinical practice patterns. *Arch. Intern. Med.* 1983; 143:1861–62.

Lundberg, G.D. Laboratory request forms (menus) that guide and teach. *J.A.M.A.* 1983; 249:3075.

Lundberg, G.D. Perseveration of laboratory test ordering: A syndrome affecting clinicians. *J.A.M.A.* 1983; 249:639.

Lusted, L. *A Study of the Efficacy of Diagnostic Radiologic Procedures: Final Report to the National Center for Health Services Research, Rockville, Md., 31 May 1977.* Rockville, Md.: National Center for Health Services Research, 1972.

Lyle, C.B., Jr., R.F. Bianchi, J.H. Harris, and Z.L. Wood. Teaching cost containment to house officers at Charlotte Memorial Hospital. *J. Med. Educ.* 1979; 54:856–62.

Mahler, D.M., R.M Veath, and V.W. Sidel. Ethical issues in informed consent: Research in medical cost containment. *J.A.M.A.* 1982; 247:481–85.

Manning, W.G. *The Use of Pathology Services: A Comparison of Fee-for-Service and a Prepaid Group Practice.* Santa Monica, Calif.: Rand Corp., January 1983. Rand Corp. Pub. R–2919–HCFA.

Manu, P., and S.E. Schwartz. Patterns of diagnostic testing in the academic setting: The influence of medical attendings' subspecialty training. *Soc. Sci. Med.* 1983; 17:1339–42.

Marcy, W.L., S.T. Miller, and R. Vander Zwaag. Modification of admission diagnostic test ordering by residents. *J. Fam. Pract.* 1981; 12:141–42.

Markel, G.A. Hospital utilization effects of case reimbursement for medical care. In Gabel, J.R., J. Taylor, N.T. Greenspan, and M.O. Blaxall, eds. *Physicians and Financial Incentives: Health Care Financing Conference Proceedings.* Washington, D.C.: Health Care Financing Administration, 1978; 95–99.

Maronde, R.F., P.V. Lee, M.M. McCarron, and S. Seibert. A study of prescribing patterns. *Med. Care.* 1971; 9:383–95.

Marquis, M.S. *Laboratory Test Ordering by Physicians: The Effect of Reimbursement Policies.* Santa Monica, Calif.: Rand Corp., August 1982. Rand Corp. Pub. R–2901–HCFA.

Martin, A.R., M.A. Wolf, L.A. Thibodeau, V. Dzau, and E.Braunwald. A trial of two strategies to modify the test-ordering behavior of medical residents. *N. Engl. J. Med.* 1980; 303:1330–36.

Martin, S.G., M. Schwartz, B.J. Whalen, et al. Impact of a mandatory second-opinion program on Medicaid surgery rates. *Med. Care.* 1982; 20:21–45.

Marton, K.I., H.C. Sox, J. Alexander, and C.E. Duisenberg. Attitudes of patients toward diagnostic tests: The case of the upper gastrointestinal series roentgenogram. *Med. Decis. Making.* 1982; 2:439–48.

Marton, K.I., H.C. Sox, J. Wasson, and C.E. Duisenberg. The clinical value of the upper gastrointestinal tract roentgenogram series. *Arch. Intern. Med.* 1980; 140:191–95.

Marton, K.I., V. Tul, and H.C. Sox. Modifying test-ordering behavior in the outpatient medical clinic: A controlled trial of two educational interventions. *Arch. Intern. Med.* 1985; 145:816–21.

McCarthy, E.G., and M.L. Finkel. Second opinion elective surgery programs: Outcome status over time. *Med. Care.* 1978; 16:984–94.

McCombs, J.S. Physician treatment decisions in a multiple treatment model: The effects of physician supply. *J. Health Econ.* 1984; 3:155–71.

McConnell, T.S., P.R. Berger, H.H. Dayton, B.E. Umland, and B.E. Skipper. Professional review of laboratory utilization. *Hum. Pathol.* 1982; 13:399–403.

McDonald, C.J., S.L. Hui, D.M. Smith, et al. Reminders to physicians from an introspective computer medical record: A two-year randomized trial. *Ann. Intern. Med.* 1984; 100:130–38.

McGowan, J.E., and M. Finland. Effects of monitoring the usage of antibiotics: An inter-hospital comparison. *South. Med. J.* 1976; 69:193–95.

McGowan, J.E., and M. Finland. Usage of antibiotics in a general hospital: Effect of requiring justification. *J. Infect. Dis.* 1974; 130:253–59.

McNeil, B.J., R. Weichselbaum, and S.G. Pauker. Fallacy of the five year survival in lung cancer. *N. Engl. J. Med.* 1978; 299:1397–401.

McNeil, B.J., B. Weichselbaum, and S.G. Pauker. Speech and survival: Tradeoffs between quality and quantity of life in laryngeal cancer. *N. Engl. J. Med.* 1981; 305:982–87.

McPhee, S.J., S.A. Chapman, L.P. Myers, S.A. Schroeder, and J.K. Leong. Lessons for teaching cost containment. *J. Med. Educ.* 1984; 59:722–29.

McPherson, K., P.M. Strong, A. Epstein, and L. Jones. Regional variations in the use of common surgical procedures; within and between England and Wales, Canada and the United States of America. *Soc. Sci. Med.* 1981; 15A:273–88.

McPherson, K., J.E. Wennberg, O.B. Hovind, and P. Clifford. Small-area variations in the use of common surgical procedures: An international comparison of New England, England, and Norway. *N. Engl. J. Med.* 1982; 307:1310–14.

Melmon, K.L., and T.F. Blaschke. The undereducated physician's therapeutic decisions. *N. Engl. J. Med.* 1983; 308:1473–74.

Menzel, P.T. *Medical Costs, Moral Choices: A Philosophy of Health Care Economics in America.* New Haven, Conn.: Yale University Press, 1983.

Mistry, F.D., and J.S. Davis. Teaching efficient and effective utilization of the clinical laboratory. *J. Med. Educ.* 1981; 56:356–58.

Mitchell, J.B., and J. Cromwell. Variations in surgery rates and the supply of surgeons. In Rothberg, D.L., ed. *Regional Variations in Hospital Use.* Lexington, Mass.: Lexington Books, 1982; 103–30.

Moore, S. Cost containment through risk-sharing by primary care physicians. *N. Engl. J. Med.* 1979; 300:1359–62.

Moore, S.H., D.P. Martin, and W.C. Richardson. Does the primary care gatekeeper control the costs of health care? Lessons from the SAFECO experience. *N. Engl. J. Med.* 1983; 309:1400–1404.

Munch, P. Economic incentives to order lab tests: Theory and evidence. In Hough, D.E.,and G.I. Misek, eds. *Socioeconomic Issues of Health.* Chicago: American Medical Assoc., 1980; 59–83.

Mushlin, A.I., and F.A. Appel. Extramedical factors in the decision to hospitalize medical patients. *Am. J. Public Health.* 1976; 66:170–72.

Myers, L.P., and S.A. Schroeder. Physician use of services for the hospitalized patient: A review, with implications for cost containment. *Milbank Mem. Fund Q.* 1981; 59:481–507.

Naisbitt, J. *Megatrends.* New York: Warner Books, 1982; 17.

Nanji, A.A. Medical grand rounds and laboratory use. *J.A.M.A.* 1983; 249:2890.

Nelson, R.B. Teaching technologic restraint: An evaluation of a single session. *Eval. Health Prof.* 1978; 1:21–28.

Newhouse, J.P., W.G. Manning, C.N. Morris, et al. Some interim results from a controlled trial of cost sharing in health insurance. *N. Engl. J. Med.* 1981; 305:1501–7.

Noie, N.E., S.M. Shortell, and M.A. Morrisey. A survey of hospital medical staffs. *Hospitals.* 1983; 57(Dec. 1):80–83.

Noren, J., T. Frazier, I. Altman, and J. DeLozier. Ambulatory medical care: A

comparison of internists and family-general practitioners. *N. Engl. J. Med.*
1980; 302:11–16.

Paris, M., J. McNemara, and M. Schwartz. Monitoring ambulatory care: Impact
of a surveillance program on clinical practice patterns in New York City. *Am.
J. Public Health.* 1980; 70:783–88.

Pauker, S.G., and J.P. Kassirer. The threshold approach to clinical decision making. *N. Engl. J. Med.* 1980; 302:1109–17.

Pauly, M.V. *Doctors and Their Workshops.* Chicago: National Bureau of Economic
Research, The University of Chicago Press, 1980.

Pauly, M.V. Medical staff characteristics and hospital costs. *J. Hum. Resour.* 1978;
13(suppl):77–111.

Pauly, M.V., and M.A. Satterthwaite. The effect of provider supply on price. In
The Target Income Hypothesis and Related Issues in Health Manpower. Washington, D.C.: Bureau of Health Manpower, Department of Health, Education
and Welfare, 1980; 26–36. DHEW publication no. (HRA) 80–27.

Penchansky, R., and D. Fox. Frequency of referral and patient characterisitcs in
group practice. *Med. Care.* 1980; 8:368–85.

Perkoff, G.T. Economic versus professional incentives for cost control. *N. Engl.
J. Med.* 1982; 307:1399–1401.

Pineault, R. The effect of prepaid group practice on physicians' utilization behavior. *Med. Care.* 1976; 14:121–36.

Ray, W.A., C.F. Federspiel, and W. Schaffner. A study of antipsychotic drug use
in nursing homes: Epidemiologic evidence suggesting misuse. *Am. J. Public
Health.* 1980; 70:485–91.

Ray, W.A., C.F. Federspiel, and W. Schaffner. Prescribing of tetracycline to children less than 8 years old. *J.A.M.A.* 1977; 237:2069–74.

Ray, W.A., W. Schaffner, and C.F. Federspiel. Persistence of improvement in
antibiotic prescribing in office practice. *J.A.M.A.* 1985; 253:1774–76.

Read, J.L., R.S. Stern, L.A. Thibodeau, D.E. Geer, Jr., and H. Klapholz. Variation in antenatal testing over time and between clinic settings. *J.A.M.A.*
1983; 249:1605–9.

Redisch, M. Physician involvement in hospital decision making. In Zubkoff,
M., I.E. Raskin, and R.S. Hanft, eds. *Hospital Cost Containment.* New York:
Prodist, 1978; 217–43.

Restuccia, J.D. The effect of concurrent feedback in reducing inappropriate hospital utilization. *Med. Care.* 1982; 20:46–62.

Rhee, S.O., R.D. Luke, and M.B. Culverwell. Influence of client/colleague dependence on physician performance in patient care. *Med. Care.* 1980;
18:829–41.

Rhyne, R.L., and S.H. Gehlback. Effects of an educational feedback strategy on
physician utilization of thyroid function panels. *J. Fam. Pract.* 1979; 8:1003–7.

Rice, T.H. The impact of changing Medicare reimbursement rates on physician-
induced demand. *Med. Care.* 1983; 21:803–15.

Rich, E.C., T.W. Crowson, and D.P. Connelly. Evidence for an informal clinical policy resulting in high use of a very-low-yield test. *Am. J. Med.* 1985; 79:577–82.

Roberts, C.J., F.G. Fowkes, W.P. Ennis, and M. Mitchell. Possible impact of audit on chest x-ray requests from surgical wards. *Lancet.* 1983; 2:446–48.

Rock, W.A., Jr., and J.E. Grogan. Demand versus need versus physician perogatives in the use of the WBC differential. *J.A.M.A.* 1983; 249:613–16.

Roemer, M.I. Bed supply and hospital utilization: A natural experiment. *Hospitals.* 1961; 35:36–42.

Rogers, F.M. *Diffusion of Innovations.* New York: Free Press, 1983.

Roos, L.L. Issues in studying ancillary services. *Soc. Sci. Med.* 1982; 16:1583–90.

Roos, L.L., Jr. Supply, workload and utilization: A population-based analysis of surgery in rural Manitoba. *Am. J. Public Health.* 1983; 73:414–21.

Roos, L.L., Jr., N.P. Roos, S.M. Cageorge, and J.P. Nicol. How good are the data: Reliability of one health care data bank. *Med. Care.* 1982; 20:266–76.

Roos, N.P. Hysterectomy: Variation in rates across small areas and across physicians' practices. *Am. J. Public Health.* 1984; 74:327–35.

Roos, N.P., and L.L. Roos, Jr. Surgical rate variations: Do they reflect the health or socioeconomic characteristics of the populations? *Med. Care.* 1982; 20:945–58.

Roos, N.P., G. Flowerdew, A. Wajda, and R.B. Tate. Variations in physicians' hospitalization practices: A population-based study in Manitoba, Canada. *Am. J. Public Health.* 1986; 76:45–51.

Rose, H., and B. Abel-Smith. *Doctors, Patients, and Pathology.* London: G. Bell and Sons, 1972. Occasional papers on Social Administration, No. 49.

Rosenblatt, R.A., and I.S. Moscovice. The physician as gatekeeper: Determinants of physicians' hospitalization rates. *Med. Care.* 1984; 22:150–59.

Rosser, W.W. Using the perception-reality gap to alter prescribing patterns. *J. Med. Educ.* 1983; 58:728–32.

Rossiter, L.F., and G.R. Wilensky. A reexamination of the use of physician services: The role of physician-initiated demand. *Inquiry.* 1983; 10:162–72.

Rothberg, D.L. Regional variations in hospital use: Introduction and overview. In Rothberg, D.L., ed. *Regional Variations in Hospital Use.* Lexington, Mass.: Lexington Books, 1982; 1–20.

Rothert, M.L., D.R. Rovner, A.S. Elstein, G.B. Holzman, M.M. Holmes, and M.M. Ravitch. Differences in medical referral decisions for obesity among family practitioners, general internists, and gynecologists. *Med. Care.* 1984; 22:42–55.

Royal College of Radiologists. Preoperative chest radiography. *Lancet.* 1979; 2:83–86.

Ruchlin, H.S., M.L. Finkel, and E.G. McCarthy. The efficacy of second-opinion consultation programs: A cost-benefit perspective. *Med. Care.* 1982; 20:3–20.

Sanazaro, P.J. Determining physicians' performance: Continuing medical education and other interacting variables. *Eval. Health Prof.* 1983; 6:197–210.

Schaffner, W., W.A. Ray, C.F. Federspiel, and W.O. Miller. Improving antibiotic prescribing in office practice: A controlled trial of three educational methods. *J.A.M.A.* 1983; 250:1728–32.

Schicke, R.K. Economic aspects of diagnostic services in health care. *Methods Inf. Med.* 1983; 22:1–3.

Schroeder, S.A. Variations in physician practice patterns: A review of medical cost implications. In Carols, E.J., D. Neuhauser, and W.B. Stason, eds. *The Physician and Cost Control.* Cambridge, Mass.: Oelgeschlager, Gunn & Hain, 1980.

Schroeder, S.A., K. Kenders, J.K. Cooper, and T.E. Piemme. Use of laboratory tests and pharmaceuticals: Variation among physicians and effect of cost audit on subsequent use. *J.A.M.A.* 1973; 225:969–73.

Schroeder, S.A., L.P. Myers, S.J. McPhee, et al. The failure of physician education as a cost containment strategy: Report of a prospective controlled trial at a university hospital. *J.A.M.A.* 1984; 252:225–30.

Schroeder, S.A., A. Schliftman, and T.E. Piemme. Variation among physicians in use of laboratory tests: Relation to quality of care. *Med. Care.* 1974; 12:709–13.

Schroeder, S.A., and J.A. Showstack. Financial incentives to perform medical procedures and laboratory tests: Illustrative models of office practice. *Med. Care.* 1978; 16:289–98.

Schwartz, J.S., S.V. Williams, J.M. Eisenberg, and D. Kitz. Effect of utilization review on physician billing [Abstract]. *Med. Decis. Making.* 1981; 1:466.

Schwartz, M., S.G. Martin, D.D. Cooper, G.M. Ljung, B.J. Whalen, and J. Blackburn. The effect of a thirty percent reduction in physician fees on Medicaid surgery rates in Massachusetts. *Am. J. Public Health.* 1981; 71:370–75.

Sherman, A.R. *Behavior Modification: Theory and Practice.* Monterey, Calif.: Brooks/Cole Pub. Co., 1973.

Sherman, H. Surveillance effects on community physician test ordering. *Med. Care.* 1984; 22:80–83.

Shortell, S.M., T.M. Wickizer, and J.R.C. Wheeler. *Hospital-Physician Joint Ventures: Results and Lessons from a National Demonstration in Primary Care.* Ann Arbor, Mich.: Health Administration Press, 1984.

Sims, P.D., D. Cabral, W. Daley, and L. Alfano. The incentive plan: An approach for modification of physician behavior. *Am. J. Public Health.* 1984; 74:150–52.

Singer, D.E., P.L. Carr, A.G. Mulley, and G.E. Thibault. Rationing intensive care: Physician responses to a resource shortage. *N. Engl. J. Med.* 1983; 309:1155–60.

Skinner, B.F. *The Behavior of Organisms.* New York: Appleton-Century, 1938.

Sloan, F., J. Mitchell, and J. Cromwell. Physician participation in state Medicaid programs. *J. Hum. Resour.* 1978; 13(suppl):211–45.

Smith, S.R. An evaluation of computerized exercise in teaching cost consciousness. *J. Med. Educ.* 1983; 58:146–48.

Smits, H.L. The PSRO in perspective. *N. Engl. J. Med.* 1981; 305:253–59.

Solomon, S. How one hospital broke its inflation fever. *Fortune.* 1979; 99:148–54.

Somers, A.R. *Health Care in Transition.* Chicago: Hospital Research and Educational Trust, 1971.

Sommers, L.S., R. Sholtz, R.M. Shepherd, and D.B. Starkweather. Physician involvement in quality assurance. *Med. Care.* 1984; 22:1115–38.

Soumerai, S.B., and J. Avorn. Efficacy and cost-containment in hospital pharmacotherapy: State of the art and future directions. *Milbank Mem. Fund Q.* 1984; 62:447–74.

Special Task Force on Professional Liability and Insurance. *Professional Liability in the 80s.* Chicago: American Medical Assoc., October 1984.

Spivey, B.E. The relation between hospital management and medical staff under a prospective-payment system. *N. Engl. J. Med.* 1984; 310:984–86.

Stein, L.S. Education of residents [Letter]. *J.A.M.A.* 1981; 246:1299.

Stoelwinder, J.U., and P.S. Clayton. Hospital organization development: Changing the focus from "better management" to "better patient care." *J. Appl. Behav. Sci.* 1978; 14:400–414.

Stolley, P.D., M.H. Becker, L. Lasagna, J.D. McEvilla, and L.M. Sloane. The relationship between physician characteristics and prescribing appropriateness. *Med. Care.* 1972; 10:17–28.

Stross, J.K., and G.G. Bole. Evaluation of a continuing education program in rheumatoid arthritis. *Arthritis Rheum.* 1980; 23:846–49.

Stross, J.K., R.G. Hiss, C.M. Watts, W.K. Davis, and R. McDonald. Continuing education in pulmonary disease for primary care physicians. *Am. Rev. Respir. Dis.* 1983; 127:739–46.

Sussman, E., P. Goodwin, and H. Rosen. Administrative change and diagnostic test use. *Med. Care.* 1984; 22:569–72.

Tatchell, M. Measuring hospital output: A review of the service mix and case mix approaches. *Soc. Sci. Med.* 1983; 17:871–83.

Thompson, R.S., H.L. Kirz, and R.A. Gold. Changes in physician behavior and cost savings associated with organizational recommendations on the use of "routine" chest x-rays and multichannel blood tests. *Prev. Med.* 1983; 12:385–96.

Tuohy, C. Does a claims monitoring system influence high-volume medical practitioners? Attitudinal data from Ontario. *Inquiry.* 1982; 19:18–33.

Uhlmann, R.F., T.S. Inui, and W.B. Carter. Patient requests and expectations. *Med. Care.* 1984; 22:681–85.

Upstate surgeons curb practices to offset soaring insurance fees. *New York Times.* 1985 May 30: B8.

Vautrain, R.L., and P.F. Griner. Physician's orders, use of nursing resources, and subsequent clinical events. *J. Med. Educ.* 1978; 53:125–28.

Vayda, E. A comparison of surgical rates in Canada and in England and Wales. *N. Engl. J. Med.* 1973; 289:1224–29.

Vayda, E., and W.R. Mindell. Variations in operative rates: What do they mean? *Surg. Clin. North Am.* 1982; 62:627–39.

Weitberg, A.B. Laboratory testing in teaching hospitals: Impact on the cost of health care. *R.I. Med. J.* 1980; 63:441–42.

Wennberg, J.E. Dealing with medical practice variations: A proposal for action. *Health Aff.* 1984; 3:6–32.

Wennberg, J.E. On patient need, equity, supplier-induced demand and the need to assess the outcome of common medical practices. *Med. Care.* 1985; 23:512–20.

Wennberg, J.E. Testimony before Senate Committee on Appropriations, Subcommittee on Labor, Health and Human Services, and Education; 19 November 1984.

Wennberg, J.E., B.A. Barnes, and M. Zubkoff. Professional uncertainty and the problem of supplier-induced demand. *Soc. Sci. Med.* 1982; 16:811–24.

Wennberg, J.E., L. Blowers, R. Parker, and A.M. Gittelsohn. Changes in tonsillectomy rates associated with feedback and review. *Pediatrics.* 1977; 59:821–26.

Wennberg, J.E., and A. Gittelsohn. Health care delivery in Maine: I. Patterns of use of common surgical procedures. *J. Maine Med. Assoc.* 1975; 66:123–30, 149.

Wennberg, J.E., and A. Gittelsohn. Small area variations in health care delivery. *Science.* 1973; 182:1102–8.

Wennberg, J.E., and A. Gittelsohn. Variations in medical care among small areas. *Sci. Am.* 1982; 246(4):120–34.

Wennberg, J.E., K. McPherson, and P. Caper. Will payment based on diagnosis related groups control hospital costs? *N. Engl. J. Med.* 1984; 311:295–300.

Wertman, B.G., S.V. Sostrin, Z. Pavlova, and G.D. Lundberg. Why do physicians order laboratory tests? A study of laboratory test request and use patterns. *J.A.M.A.* 1980; 243:2080–82.

White, R.E., B.B. Quimby, B.J. Skipper, and G.D. Webster. Cost of residents' decisions on actual patients and in simulated encounters. *J. Med. Educ.* 1984; 59:834–35.

Whiting-O'Keefe, Q.E., C. Henke, and D.W. Simborg. Choosing the correct unit of analysis in medical care experiments. *Med. Care.* 1984; 22:1101–14.

Wilensky, G.R., and L.F. Rossiter. The relative importance of physician-induced demand for medical care. *Milbank Mem. Fund Q.* 1983; 61:252–77.

Williams, R.L., and P.M. Chen. Controlling the rise in cesarean section rates by the dissemination of information from vital records. *Am. J. Public Health.* 1983; 73:863–67.

Williams, S.V., and J.M. Eisenberg. Decreasing diagnostic test utilization. *J. Gen. Intern. Med.* 1986; 1:8–13.

Williams, S.V., J.M. Eisenberg, D.S. Kitz, et al. Teaching cost-effective diagnostic test use to medical students. *Med. Care.* 1984; 22:535–42.

Williams, S.V., J.M. Eisenberg, L.A. Pascale, and D.S. Kitz. Physicians' perceptions about unnecessary diagnostic testing. *Inquiry.* 1982; 19:363–70.

Williams, S.V., J.M. Eisenberg, L. Poyss, and S.I. Rubin. Decreasing diagnostic test utilization [Abstract]. *Clin. Res.* 1981; 29:337A.

Williamson, J.W., D.M. Barr, E. Fee, et al. *Teaching Quality Assurance and Cost Containment in Health Care: A Faculty Guide.* San Francisco: Jossey-Bass, 1982.

Williamson, J.W., D.M. Barr, E. Fee, et al. *Teaching Quality Assurance and Cost Containment in Health Care: A Faculty Guide.* San Francisco: Jossey-Bass, 1982.

Wilson, C.W., J.A. Banks, R.E. Mapes, and S.M. Korte. Pattern of prescribing in general practice. *Br. Med. J.* 1963; 2:604–7.

Wilson, G.A., C.J. McDonald, and G.P. McCabe, Jr. The effect of immediate access to a computerized medical record on physician test ordering: A controlled clinical trial in the emergency room. *Am. J. Public Health.* 1982; 72:698–702.

Winickoff, R.N., K.L. Coltin, M.M. Morgan, R.C. Buxbaum, and G.O. Barnett. Improving physician performance through peer comparison feedback. *Med. Care.* 1984; 22:527–34.

Winkler, J.D., K.N. Lohr, and R.H. Brook. Persuasive communication and medical technology assessment. *Arch. Intern. Med.* 1985; 145:314–17.

Wong, E.T., M.M. McCarron, and S.T. Shaw, Jr. Ordering of laboratory tests in a teaching hospital: Can it be improved? *J.A.M.A.* 1983; 249:3076–80.

Wyszewianski, L., J.R.C. Wheeler, and A. Donabedian. Market-oriented cost-containment strategies and quality of care. *Milbank Mem. Fund Q.* 1982; 60:518–50.

Yelin, E.H., C.J. Henke, J.S. Kramer, et al. A comparison of the treatment of rheumatoid arthritis in health maintenance organizations and fee-for-service practices. *N. Engl. J. Med.* 1985; 312:962–67.

Young, D.W. An aid to reducing unnecessary investigations. *Br. Med. J.* 1980; 281:1610–11.

Young, D.W., and R.B. Saltman. Medical practice, case mix, and cost containment: A new role for the attending physician. *J.A.M.A.* 1982; 247:801–5.

Young, D.W., and R.B. Saltman. Preventive medicine for hospital costs. *Harv. Bus. Rev.* 1983; 61:126–33.

Zelnio, R.N. The interaction among the criteria physicians use when prescribing. *Med. Care.* 1982; 20:277–85.

Zuidema, G.D. The problem of cost containment in teaching hospitals: The Johns Hopkins experience. *Surgery.* 1980; 87:41–45.

Index